FLEXIBLE DIETING
FOR VEGANS

The vegan athlete's guide to eating the
foods you love while improving your
physique and performance

DANI TAYLOR

TABLE OF CONTENTS

1 INTRODUCTION

I grew up in a household of junk food –
not the normal amounts of junk food that kids
sometimes get away with, but solely junk
food. Hamburger Helper was a regular dinner,
as were fried bologna and egg cups; I ate hot
dogs cold out of the package, and until I was a
teenager, I actually thought mashed potatoes
came out of a box of flakes that you mixed with
milk and margarine.

What were vegetables? Well, vegetables,
to me, were sad, frozen, diced bits of lima beans,
corn and carrots that were often side dishes to

overcooked pork chops. At restaurants, my siblings and I would often eat the jelly packets on the table while we waited for our mozzarella sticks and chicken finger meals. I vividly remember a server bringing us bowls of blue cheese dressing to eat with a spoon on more than one occasion. Have I painted a gross enough picture for you? To me, this was perfectly normal.

Not surprisingly, I was overweight.

I became a vegetarian at the age of eight, after seeing a lobster, whom I had been playing with all day in a kiddie pool in the basement, dropped in a pot of boiling water for dinner, and I lost it. I cried so hard and kicked and screamed. I didn't understand how anyone could do such a thing, let alone my own parents! It was that day that a light went off over my head and I realized that "chicken nuggets" were actually made out of chickens!

My parents were not pleased, but I was determined not to eat meat and for the next 8 years or so, I basically lived on a diet of dairy and various bread products. (Think pizza and grilled cheese. Lots of pizza and grilled cheese.) I became more and more overweight each year topping out at 210 pounds at the age of 17.

That same year, as I was doing research for an English paper about vegetarianism, I stumbled across a website that explained the connections between the dairy and egg industries and the meat industry. I was shocked! It had never occurred to me that dairy cows and egg-laying chickens were treated so poorly and eventually slaughtered to become the "foods" that I had abstained from for so long.

Never once did it occur to me that the meat industry relied upon the dairy and egg industries to keep sending them the dairy and egg animals that could no longer produce enough product to be useful. With absolutely no prior knowledge of veganism, and not knowing a single vegan, I went vegan overnight.

A strange thing began to happen after I went vegan. Even on a crappy teenage diet of plain bagels, French fries and soda, I was dropping weight and quickly. Without even noticing, I had lost 30 pounds in a few months.

For the first time in my life, it began to occur to me that I actually had some control over my body, when all this time I believed I was just genetically pre-destined to be overweight.

I began working out and researching nutrition to learn more about healthy foods. I had my first mango and avocado and so many other cool foods I had never seen before. I learned how to cook properly. I continued to drop weight steadily.

I then began tracking what I ate religiously to learn more about my body and see what worked and what didn't. I read books about dieting and "Eating Clean" and "super foods" and "detoxes".

I wanted to be the most pristine eater I could be.

I began lifting weights, and I fell in love with it. Trainers were happy to teach me how to lift, but they had no idea how to help me when it came to my diet. I heard over and over again that I couldn't possibly get enough protein to build the muscle that I was looking to build.

Frustrated, I took to the internet and kept researching on my own. What were the non-vegan weight lifters eating? Surely, I could find a way to veganize it, right? Well, I tried, and I failed. I could not figure out how to get that much protein while controlling my carbohydrates and fats. It was incredibly frustrating, and I was spinning my wheels.

I finally hit the jackpot, when I found an online trainer who was vegan! She had an incredible body, strong and fit, and seemed to be exactly what I was looking for. I signed up with her immediately. Upon receiving my meal plan, I was nervous, because following a meal plan was very new to me. It seemed quite boring and the amount of food was small, but you have to suffer to succeed, right?

Well, that's what I thought, so I followed it to a T.

I did get some decent results physically, but mentally, I was becoming obsessed with food. I would dream about my next meal all the time, and when it came, it was so bland that it wasn't even worth it.

I had a cheat meal on Sundays, and I lived for this meal and all of the options that I could choose from for that meal. Sometimes, the options even overwhelmed me to the point of not knowing what to eat. It started small, but over several months, Sundays turned into an all-out binge fest, and I would vow every week to be even stricter with my diet.

All week long, I would be hungry and tired and dream of food and on the weekend, I would eat until my stomach hurt and the guilt and fear would set in. I had undone a week's worth of work and so on and so forth . . .

This spiral continued until I had a full-blown eating disorder and had to take a giant step back from the fitness world for several years for my own health.

Reading this, you may see several red flags that I too should have seen. But I was 18 years old and had no idea what to look for in a good coach, and I assumed if someone had the body I wanted, that they would know how to help me get it (that's a topic for another book entirely!). While it's easy to say, "This would never happen to me. I would never let it get to that point," I assure you that it happens all the time and I see it in my inbox daily.

This is an incredibly common story told by both men and women in the fitness industry, some new and some veterans. Some people are so caught up in this food obsession cycle that they can't even see how unhealthy it is. It's the new normal. The idea of "eating clean" as often as they can, and inevitably bingeing (sometimes in a planned fashion), is so commonplace that it's sad.

Often times, the health industry is anything but.

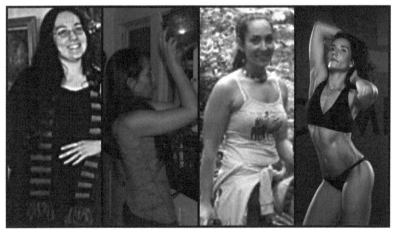

From left to right: (1) December 2003, a new vegan already down 10 pounds from a starting weight of 210 pounds. (2) July 2008. Obsessed with clean eating, on a strict meal plan and always anxious about food. (3) October 2009. Having intense binging episodes and absolutely hating myself for it. (4) July 2014. 2 days before competing and placing first in my class. Utilizing flexible dieting through my whole contest prep.

Alongside the general fitness community is the vegan community, which is so divided by food choices that in many ways, it is worse than the mainstream fitness community. How many variations of the vegan diet are there? Gluten Free. Soy Free. HCLF. Raw Vegan. Fruitarian. Oil Free. Sugar Free. Keto Vegan. I could go on forever . . .

Everyone is entitled to eat whatever they choose, of course. Where the problem lies, is that some people get so caught up in eating the cleanest, most whole-food based, least refined, most organic, etc., etc., ad nauseum, that they become obsessed with being the purest eater in the world, and oftentimes, build very unhealthy relationships with foods and "fall off the wagon," the same way I did many years ago. Ironically, this often leads to poorer health, worse performance, and an inability to reach aesthetic physique goals as well.

I am here to say that there is another way.

When I finally felt able to step back into the fitness industry, I decided I was going to try something else. I was going to try and eat roughly the same number of calories, carbohydrates, protein, and fat that I was getting results with previously, but I was going to do it by eating foods that I actually enjoyed. I would just see what happened. And thus began my journey into flexible dieting.

Now, I am by no stretch of the imagination implying that I invented flexible dieting (also often called IIFYM, If It Fits Your Macros or Macro Tracking). But at the time, there was no one else that I knew approaching their diet this way. This is simply the approach that worked for me nearly twelve years ago, and it seemed like people all over the world, vegan or not, were realizing that it worked for them as well.

I believe the term was actually coined in a bodybuilding.com forum, but regardless, the principles are the same: **Eat what you want to hit your properly planned macronutrient requirements, and you will achieve results.**

Long story made very short: You can work toward your fitness and physique goals without driving yourself crazy. You can get decently lean without turning down social events. You can have abs and eat vegan cookies, in moderation and—be GUILT FREE with proper planning—right alongside your broccoli and tempeh. The following is a detailed book to help you learn how.

2 WHAT IS FLEXIBLE DIETING?

Flexible Dieting, sometimes called IIFYM (an acronym for "If It Fits Your Macros"), is all about freedom of food choices. It's about eating in a flexible manner that allows you to still live your life. It's about eating in a sustainable way, to get or keep the body and performance that you want, while creating as little anxiety and obsession around food as possible. Whether your goal is to run a marathon, enter a powerlifting meet, get shredded for a bodybuilding show, pack on lean muscle, or drop 15 pounds, you can utilize flexible dieting while living a vegan lifestyle.

At its most basic level, flexible dieting is about hitting your daily nutrition targets with whatever foods you choose. In a way, that's really all it is, but on a larger scale, it is so much more than that.

Flexible dieting is a way to create and maintain an eating style that allows you to reach your goals while actually adding to your quality of living rather than taking away from it.

I think that we can all agree that being strong and relatively lean is something that most people want. So is having a social life and enjoying the pleasures that delicious foods bring. Flexible dieting is about not sacrificing one for the other. If you have come to a point where you resent your eating style for any reason, you are not going to achieve your goals. You will need to change something if you ever want to make real progress and maintain it.

At its very core, flexible dieting is about "hitting your macros," but it is ultimately a way out of dietary restriction regardless of your fitness goals. **It is not just another set of numbers to obsess about.** There would be nothing flexible about that.

It is not something that is learned overnight, and like anything else, it will take a little experimentation and a lot of practice to see what works best for *you* and your lifestyle.

What doesn't bend, breaks, and it's not called flexible dieting for nothing! Your eating style needs to flow with your lifestyle and since life often throws us curveballs, you need to be flexible enough with your eating plan to allow for this. For many fitness enthusiasts and die-hard meal planners, this is the hardest thing to embrace. You don't need to be absolutely dead-on with everything you eat one hundred percent of the time.

PRO TIP: Nutrition labels can be off by up to 20%[1], so the belief that you ever *really* know exactly what you're eating is an idea that you need to let go of right this minute. However, that doesn't mean that we can't get *really* close, and do so without obsessing.

WHY FLEXIBLE DIETING?

If you have fitness or physique goals, what you eat is going to play a huge role in whether you achieve them or not. Eating improperly can make exercise nearly useless and you end up scratching your head wondering what is wrong with you. Nine times out of ten, the problem lies in the diet.

Most people have a hunch that the problem in their progress has something to do with what they're putting (or not putting) in their mouths, and eventually take to their diet and "clean it up," often cutting out things like refined carbs, sugars, overt fats, gluten, etc.

Maybe they hire a diet coach who makes them a meal plan full of clean foods that will get them to their goals. Maybe they decide to do a "juice cleanse" or a "sugar detox." Will these methods work? Maybe. It's possible, but will they last? Almost certainly not.

Unless you plan on eating out of Tupperware every time you leave your house for the rest of your life, you are likely going to lose your results when you reach your goal and slip up on your new eating habits, or go back to your normal way of eating. Can a juice fast last forever? No, and nor should it.

By learning how to eat flexibly, you give yourself a set of tools that you can use for the rest of your life, at any given moment. Does this mean you have to eat *exactly* X grams of protein, carbs, fat and fiber, every day forever? NO! How would that be flexible?! You have some wiggle room. How close you need to get to your macros will be determined by the precision needed for your particular goals, which we will get into later.

In my own personal experience, myself and many others I have worked with have been able to develop healthy relationships with foods, neither afraid of it *nor* obsessed with it, while both working towards our athletic goals and actually living our lives.

WHAT'S WRONG WITH A MEAL PLAN?

I have written meal plans for people for many years, and I absolutely do believe they have their place and can be incredibly helpful in many situations. I work hard to make my meal plans very personalized, varied, delicious to help my clients achieve their goals. I ask clients what foods they like, what foods they miss, and never say, "Well, you can't have X anymore." But this is certainly not true for all, or even most coaches—not to toot my own horn, but true custom meal plans are far more work than most people are willing to put in.

There are many, many, *many* fitness professionals out there, handing out meal plans with the same 5-7 foods on them, every day for months, low to no carbs, eating 6 small meals three hours apart, and giving the exact same plan to every man and every woman. These are dangerous and, dare I say, stupid diets that do not take into consideration much about a person's lifestyle, and they disregard the client's mental welfare entirely.

As a starting point, I feel that a (well designed) meal plan can be a great way to learn portion sizes and what a balanced day of food intake looks like. Clients learn which carb sources make them feel good and which ones make them feel bloated. They learn what the proper amount of protein feels like and what certain kinds of meals do for their training sessions.

As the meal plans change (which they should as progress is made) they can also see how it changes and why. Meal plans, with proper explanations, can basically build a road map for someone wanting to learn what to eat for his or her goals, and they can be a hugely valuable teaching tool.

Serious athletes can also benefit from meal plans because it gives them one less thing to think about so that they can dedicate more of their focus to training. Also, the more serious the athlete, the more fine-tuned the plans can be as well to really nail nutrient timing and supplementation needs. With a meal plan in hand, they can go on autopilot and crush their sport of choice.

However, there comes a point where a meal plan isn't going to cut it. One cannot be expected to live on a meal plan forever, nor should they.

The client will get bored, and will eventually feel trapped by their program, even if it is food they usually enjoy. There is a strong correlation between people who diet "rigidly", via a meal plan for too long and increased disordered eating behaviors, mood disturbances, and excessive concern with body image.[2] I think most people who have tried to live on a meal plan for an extended period of time likely know exactly what I am referring to.

Even when a coach *wants* to implement a variety of foods, one person cannot possibly fulfill every craving and desire that every client

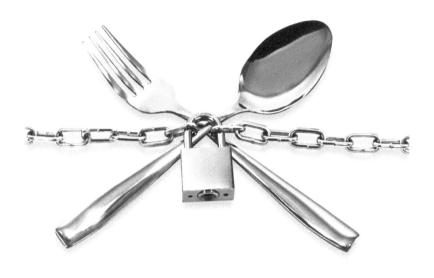

has, because they are different people, with different tastes and preferences. Most importantly, the client should ultimately learn how to make these changes on their own to satisfy their own wants, so that they can live their lives on their own terms without always needing a coach to hold their hand for the rest of their lives.

What happens when you're invited out to dinner and nothing on your meal plan is on the menu? Do you bring Tupperware and eat from that at the table? Go hungry? Completely fly off the handle and say, "Screw it" and eat everything in sight? What do you do at social events? Vacations? Holidays? Avoiding all festivities for the sake of a meal plan is a terrible way to live, especially long term, and I don't wish that on anyone.

If you have a good coach who wants to see you succeed, the end goal should be to learn how to eat for your lifestyle on your own. This can take a long time, and that's ok. But if you ask your coach a question about your plan and they can't explain why it is set up the way it is, they will not be helping you learn how to fend for yourself once you are no longer with them.

If I coach someone well enough, eventually they will be able to create their meal programs on their own and they won't need me anymore! To me, that's the marker of success with a client.

Once someone has the skill of flexible dieting in his or her back pocket, they are always armed for success, no matter the occasion—and they still get to partake in the joys of living!

PERCENTAGE-BASED MACRO SPLITS ARE NOT THE ANSWER

Ratios and percentages are a way that many people are describing their diets these days. People often say things like "I eat 50/30/20" or "80/10/10" or what have you. These are percentages of macronutrients; for example, 50% carbs, 30% protein and 20% fat.

The reason that I strongly dislike these kinds of dietary descriptions is that it tells me virtually nothing about a person's diet. That person could be eating 800 calories a day or 3000 calories a day; 50/30/20 doesn't give me any clue to that, and those are incredibly different diets.

Eating 50% carbs on an 800-calorie-per-day diet is only 100g of carbs, whereas on a 3000-calorie-a-day diet it is 375g of carbs. That's an enormous difference, which illustrates how little this percentage breakdown tells us. A percentage of an unknown number is arbitrary and pointless.

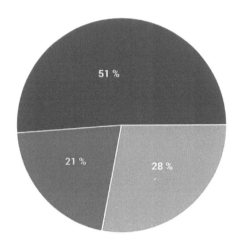

	Total	Goal
▪ Carbohydrates	51 %	50 %
▪ Fat	21 %	20 %
▪ Protein	28 %	30 %

This graph tells me very little about what someone actually eats.

Another reason that I don't like percentage-based diets is that it encourages this idea that there is a magical ratio of carbs to protein to fat, and there isn't. Ratios don't matter; absolute numbers matter and they are different for everyone.

Each human will have a different number of grams of protein and fat they require to function properly, while their caloric needs may go up and down. By simply following a percentage-based split, if caloric requirements go up, they may be wasting calories on more protein than they need when it may be much better allocated towards carbohydrates.

"I DON'T *DO* MACROS"

This is a phrase I have heard time and time again: "I don't *do* macros." Well, do you eat food? What do you think that food is made up of? **Macros!**

If you eat food, you do macros.

Just because you don't count them, does not make you somehow immune to the fact your food contains protein, carbs and fats. Someone once said, "Saying you don't do macros, is like saying you don't do gravity." You're eating macros whether you count them or not.

"CLEAN EATING" AND WHY IT NEEDS TO STOP

"I eat clean." – What does that even mean?

I can guarantee that whatever it means to you, is likely something different from what it means to the next person. There is no agreed-upon list of clean and unclean foods, and there never will be. It is an arbitrary word generally used to make people feel good or bad about their food choices.

Take for example, the vegan community. There are many people who would say gluten or even grains are unclean foods, but many Eat to Live-ers would strongly disagree. Macrobiotic vegans would say that soy is a clean food, but many vegans would say soy is a processed or dirty food. Some would say fruit isn't a clean food because it has too much sugar, while there are fruitarian groups who say fruit is basically the *only* clean food.

Do you see where I am going with this? The term "clean food," means literally nothing and there is no way to quantify it. Any word that gives morality to a person based on how healthy certain foods are and tries to make other, less-healthy foods (and the people who eat them) feel bad about it, isn't something I see a need for.

I went vegan for ethical reasons only, and I know that others have found their own unique paths to veganism. Regardless of how you got here, I am glad you're here. We're all on the same side, fighting for the same things. So, please, for the love of god, stop insulting other vegan's food choices. If it's vegan, we're all good.

AREN'T WHOLE FOODS BETTER FOR YOU?

You'd be hard pressed to find someone who can tell you, with a straight face, that an Oreo is just as good for you as broccoli. And I am certainly not about to be that person. What I will say is that we're not here to demonize or glorify any particular foods. If your macronutrients are set up properly, you will likely be eating a lot of whole foods to hit that goal, and if you don't, you will likely be pretty miserable, because eating mostly healthy foods makes us feel pretty good!

For example, I could hit my macro goals today by eating nothing but plain Boca Burgers, Un-frosted Pop Tarts, and some Fiber One (as demonstrated in a loose study by Dr. Mark Haub called "The Twinkie Diet"[3]).

I could. So why wouldn't I?

Just because we are not assigning titles to food such as clean and dirty, does not mean we should throw the baby out with the bath water. We should not disregard a century of scientific literature that overwhelmingly states that higher fruit, vegetable, grains, and beans consumption leads to improved health markers and a longer, healthier life. Basically, we're not reinventing the wheel here. We are simply remapping the way that wheel gets where it is going.

It would also be very little physical food and I would be very hungry all day long. I would rather have full plates of seitan, kale, whole grain bread with peanut butter and jelly and some buffalo style Morning Star Farms Strips at dinner.

Whole fruits and veggies are nutritionally dense, meaning they have a lot of nutrients per gram, and are typically not calorically dense, meaning they have few calories per gram, and they are great to eat when cutting or dieting, because you get a lot of food, for few calories.

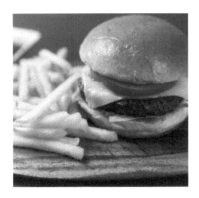
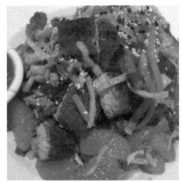

VEGGIE BURGER AND FRIES
FROM RED ROBIN

THAI TEMPEH SALAD
FROM VEGGIE GRILL

714 CALORIES	700 CALORIES
86 GRAMS CARBS	87 GRAMS CARBS
29 G FAT GRAMS	30 FAT GRAMS
30 G PROTEIN GRAMS	31 G PROTEIN GRAMS

Calorically dense foods, or foods that have a lot of calories per gram, are often seen as bad, but that's not necessarily the case. Nuts, seeds, avocados, whole grains and beans are all fairly calorically dense. So are cookies, ice cream and potato chips.

Let's imagine that you're a skinny young guy with a speedy metabolism, desperately trying to gain weight on 5,000-6,000 calories a day. Now imagine trying to do it with whole foods only.

For this young ectomorph, I imagine that would be really hard, especially since my people in his position generally have a hard time eating enough food anyway. Add to that a constantly full and bloated feeling, and he's probably going to fail. So, for him, it would be beneficial to incorporate some refined carbohydrates and processed foods to get a lot of calories without being very uncomfortable. You need to look at things on a case-by-case basis.

There is a lot of food shaming in the vegan *and* fitness world and it is one of my biggest pet peeves. There is no morality in your vegan food choices, and what I mean by that is that eating whole foods doesn't make you "good" or "pure" and unhealthy/processed foods don't make you "bad". There is no need to attach your self-worth to the types of foods that you eat. Eating foods you love, in a specific way I will teach you here today, leaves absolutely no reason for even a hint of guilt.

WHAT IS DIFFERENT ABOUT BEING VEGAN?

You may be wondering, "What does any of this have to do with being vegan?" Honestly, very little. Being vegan makes little difference in flexible dieting, which is part of the magic of it. Anyone, vegan or not, can be a flexible dieter.

There are a few key differences I've found in my practice, however.

The number one difference that I have found in my time coaching vegans is that, in general, we can eat more. Our maintenance level of calories seems to be higher than our omnivorous counterparts. Now, this is just anecdotal, and I have no scientific studies to back this up, but I have found it to be the case over and over again. I suspect that it has to do with our fiber intake being higher than non-vegans, and fiber is largely undigested, but again, it's just a theory. But for this reason, I think most calorie calculators are pretty much useless for most vegans.

The second difference in being a vegan who practices any version of IIFYM are the protein sources. You knew we had to go there in a vegan book about nutrition, didn't you?

I know I just told you that you can eat basically whatever you want to reach your macronutrient goals, and in a sense, you can! As long as you hit your goals, that is. However, when determining your macronutrient goals, most vegans will find that the protein goal is higher than what they are used to, and that's ok! You can tweak things to fit your lifestyle, and it's all about learning the skill.

All vegan protein sources, unlike many non-vegan protein sources (like chicken or egg white), also come with some additional carbohydrates and/or fats, so there is definitely a bit of a learning period required for hitting this number, whatever it may be for you. So, while a non-vegan can easily add 30g protein and zero grams of carbohydrate by eating a can of tuna, a vegan would likely add several grams of carbs and/or fat using a vegan source.

WHAT FLEXIBLE DIETING IS NOT

One of the biggest critiques of flexible dieting is that many people use it as a way to eat junk food all day and convince themselves it's for their health. Some say that it may work for physique goals but that it doesn't take a person's overall health into consideration. I don't believe this to be necessarily true.

Flexible dieting is not about cramming as much "junk" food into your day as possible. There are definitely people who do this, and I think they are taking the term, "If it fits your macros" a little too literally.

Yes, as long as you're not on a serious cut, you can probably work a treat into your plans every single day! But that doesn't mean that you get to eat nothing but processed foods and never eat anything green.

Don't get me wrong, as demonstrated above, it *can* be true, but **flexible dieting is all about what you make of it.** And this is where good ole common sense comes in to play.

I would like to think this goes without saying, but I know that there *are* some people out there just thrilled with the idea that I have given them permission to eat Oreos and protein powder all day and promised them abs as a result. That is not what I've said at all.

I think most of us understand the value of fresh vegetables, fruits, grains, legumes, nuts and seeds. They are loaded with vitamins, minerals, antioxidants, phytonutrients, and fiber. They make us feel good, they keep us "regular," and they keep us full. By all means, you should make

What Flexible Dieting Looks Like

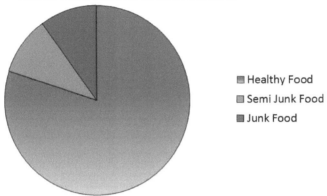

- Healthy Food
- Semi Junk Food
- Junk Food

What People Think Flexible Dieting Looks Like

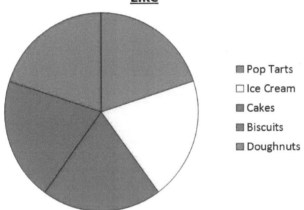

- Pop Tarts
- Ice Cream
- Cakes
- Biscuits
- Doughnuts

these foods the majority of your diet (and you will probably have to if your macros are set up properly).

But, the point is, if there is something less healthy that you're craving once in a while, or you like to have a little dessert after dinner, as long as you account for it in your daily totals, it will do **no** damage to achieving your goals; not a damn thing.

Contrary to what many would expect, it has been shown that flexible dieters actually have consistently healthier vitamin and mineral intake than "clean eaters" or people who live on a rigid meal plan.

When you think about it, it makes sense that someone eating the same half dozen foods over and over again would be very high in some vitamins, but pretty low in others. By utilizing flexible dieting to incorporate more variety into the types of foods a person eats, they also are getting a wider variety of vitamins and minerals as well.

To reiterate, flexible dieting exists as a way to enjoy a variety of foods, and to enjoy friends, family, social occasions, and eating foods you actually like, without having an anxiety attack, or flying off the handle. It is not an excuse to banish all nutrient-dense foods from your diet. Eat your veggies.

3 WHAT ARE MACROS?

"Macro" is short for macronutrients. Macronutrients, however, are what give our bodies the energy to carry out life's functions, and to create tissue in the body. They are carbohydrates, fats, proteins, and to a degree, fiber. These macronutrients contain calories, or energy.

Before we jump into explanations for each macro, I want to touch upon calories. There has been much confusion in the community over whether to track calories, or to track macros. It is important to know that each macro has a set number of calories. **If you are tracking macros, you are also tracking calories.**

MACRONUTRIENTS

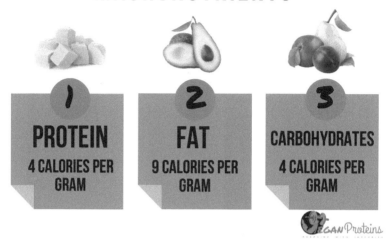

PROTEIN

Protein is the hot button for nearly any vegan, and with good reason. For as long as you've been a vegan, you have probably been poked and prodded by everyone and their brother about how you can possibly sustain life when you get no protein.

Obviously, we know that there are a lot of myths about vegans and protein, and we're all here and alive and well, and obviously we're not protein deficient. I believe that you can get enough protein, as a vegan, without much thought. If you're a sedentary person, all you need to do is eat a variety of foods and ensure that you eat enough calories to be sure you are getting enough protein to live.

But if you're reading this book you want to do more than just live, right?

When you take on an athletic endeavor (which I'm assuming most reading this book are currently doing!), your protein intake needs to change, and it becomes more critical to ensure you're getting enough of it. With planning, many people can still do this with whole foods, but there is also no shame in supplementing whether that is with a plant-based protein powder, or by eating higher protein foods like seitan, tofu or an analog food like Beyond Meat.

Many are quick to point at a vegan who supplements and say that they need supplements because their vegan diet is lacking. It's important to remember that nearly all athletes supplement in one way or another, so being vegan has nothing to do with it, rather it's the higher demands being placed on their bodies by athletic endeavors.

Proteins are made up of amino acids, which we know are in almost every food. And while you don't have to worry about food combining to make "complete" proteins, as was once believed in the 1970s[4], there are certain amino acids that are more important to muscular growth and repair than others (namely leucine[5]) so it is important to ensure that you're getting enough.

Your skeletal muscles are made up almost entirely of protein and water, and every time you work out, you break down those muscle fibers and then amino acids repair and rebuild them and make them stronger.

When your main goal is to be leaner or lose body fat, protein is a particularly important macronutrient. The reason for this is that the body actually burns energy (calories) when digesting protein, roughly 20-30 percent of the calories, in fact, in a process called thermogenesis.[6] Keeping protein relatively high while in a fat loss phase also helps to keep you satiated and decreases the likelihood of muscle loss.[7]

This doesn't mean you can eat all protein and only protein. Eating too much protein can cause fat gain just like overeating any other macronutrient does, although not quite to the same degree. [8] Eating more protein than you require doesn't mean you will gain more muscle. **Just because enough is good, that doesn't mean that more equals better.**[9]

CARBOHYDRATES

Carbohydrates are your body's first choice for fuel. Carbohydrates give you energy, and if you're an athletic person, trying to hit your workouts hard every day and reach a goal, you *need* energy! Carbohydrates also provide fuel for your brain, which as far as I can see, is a pretty important organ to keep in tip-top working order. Have you ever heard of the low-carb brain fog? Carbs are not the enemy here. The key is the right amount of carbs timed appropriately.

Under-eating carbohydrates empties your glycogen stores (consider these your human gasoline tank), which is your body's first source of energy during exercise lasting more than thirty seconds. When your body goes to use them for fuel, and there's nothing there many people think your body begins burning fat for fuel; in a perfect world, maybe. In fact, your body begins to use both fat and muscle for energy, breaking your muscle down into amino acids and using them for fuel, as well as your fat.[10] Kind of seems counterproductive to your workout, no?

On the flipside, overeating carbohydrates, like any other macronutrient will lead to weight gain, in the form of building new tissue. How much of a surplus you consume, combined with the manner in which you train, will determine how much of that is fat and how much is muscle. But grossly overeating carbs will almost certainly result in fat gain, as our bodies are only capable of building so much muscle in a certain time frame, without the use of anabolic drugs.

SLOW DIGESTING CARBS VS. SUGARY CARBS

Carbs get a bad rap all around, but they are absolutely necessary, just like the other macronutrients. The problem is that when people think "carbs," the often think of crackers, chips, cookies, candy and soda. These foods are *very* calorically dense and incredibly easy to overeat (did you know a serving size of chips, is like . . . 13 chips? Who is eating 13 chips? No one. That's my point.) and overeating anything beyond what our metabolisms are capable of using, be it bananas or vegan ice cream will cause weight gain.

But both fast-digesting and slow-digesting carbs have their place! For example, if you're headed into an intense training session and you haven't eaten in a while and all you had on you was oatmeal and Skittles (or dates—also a fast digesting carb), I would say eat the Skittles! You need that energy instantly, and that's what a fast digesting carb will give you.

Now, if you're headed into a long work meeting and know you won't be able to eat for the next several hours, eat the oatmeal—it will keep you feeling full for longer due to the fiber making it digest more slowly.

All carbs, be they fast or slow, jelly beans or quinoa, are broken down into sugar in the body.[11] At what pace is really the question. But the fact of the matter is that if you are eating within your caloric and macronutrient goals, getting enough fiber daily, and training regularly, eating some sugary, or "empty" carbs is not going to inhibit your progress at all, and at certain times, can even be beneficial.[12]

Basically, what I'm saying is if you prefer white rice over brown rice, just eat the white rice!

Generally speaking, carbs are the most easily manipulated macronutrient to tweak when either building or cutting—this is the first number to play with.

FAT

Fat is the most calorically dense macronutrient with 9 calories per gram; many people are terrified of it. Anyone remember Susan Powter yelling into crowds "It's the fat that makes you fat!" during daytime infomercials?

No?

Clearly, I'm dating myself.

Anyway, fat, like carbs, gets a bad rap because people tend to overeat it! Have you ever measured an actual serving of peanut butter? It's probably *much* smaller than you think. It's only 32g, by the way.

At 9 calories per gram, it is very easy to overeat, but it is in no way inherently bad.

Fat plays a vital role in our hormone balance, which is particularly important when dieting or cutting calories when hormones tend to shift.

Fat also allows us to absorb fat-soluble vitamins A, D, E and K, which serve many functions, not the least of which are healthy skin and hair.[13]

Essential fatty acids, which are types of fats that we need to get from our food because our bodies do not produce them on their own, help with brain and tissue development, act as anti-inflammatories, and strengthen the immune system.[13]

Did I mention they're delicious? They are incredibly satiating, despite usually being eaten in fairly small amounts. They help "tide you over" while dieting and they are also a *great* way to increase calories easily when going through a muscle building phase.

This is one place where I will clearly say that some fats are healthier than others and some are better avoided. I'm not saying never ever, ever have something with trans-fat, but I would avoid it when possible and definitely try to get the vast majority of your fat from non-hydrogenated sources, and be sure to get your Essential Fatty Acids in by eating foods such as flaxseed or by taking a high quality algae oil supplement.

FIBER

Fiber is technically a type of carbohydrate, but it acts quite differently than other carbs. Unlike starchy or sugary carbohydrates, fiber is not entirely digested by the body, although it can be broken down into short chain fatty acids in the gut and encourages good digestive flora.

As we all know, fiber keeps you "regular," and that's a good thing. The daily recommendation for fiber is about 35g a day for men and 25g a day for women. As vegans, most of us sit back and laugh at this. Yeah, for breakfast maybe! You'd be hard pressed to find a vegan that doesn't reach these fiber goals, even "junk food vegans." However, there is another end of the spectrum though, and that is eating *too much* fiber.

Your body can typically handle the amount of fiber that it's accustomed to, so "too much" will vary from person to person. However, while fiber acts as a broom that helps sweep waste through us, too much fiber can actually clog up the pipes, so to speak.

Too much fiber can lead to bloating and digestive discomfort, but more alarming than that, it can contribute to mineral deficiencies (like iron, which athletes need more of) by lowering absorption rates. Also, just as an aside, since fiber mostly goes right through you, it cuts in to the amount of carbohydrates you can actually absorb and use for energy.

My theory is that a vegan's tendency to eat far more fiber than the Standard American Diet plays a large part in why vegans seem to be able to eat more overall calories—but again, that's just a theory.

4 GETTING STARTED

I suppose this is the biggest question and the mystery that stops many people from trying flexible dieting. Many people believe that there is a magical set of macro numbers that will transform their bodies. And there very well may be certain macros that will transform *your* body—but they are going to be very individual to the person. Believe me, it would make my job much easier if it were as simple as applying a math equation to everyone and then everyone would have their perfect macros for the rest of their lives, but it isn't. There is *some* math though! So, let's get down to it.

FINDING YOUR MAINTENANCE CALORIES

Google "How many calories should I eat?" and you will find endless calculators, each giving you a different caloric number, and leaving you completely confused and lost, and not knowing what to believe. While these types of calculators can serve their purpose in certain situations, they are still ballpark figures and often with a very wide range, so I suggest sparing yourself the headache and not relying on them.

Although humans have the same basic physiology, you are very individual in many ways! You have your own unique lifestyle, sleeping patterns, body fat percentage, age, hormone levels, energy patterns, metabolism, eating habits, etc. and no calculator on the Internet will take all of that into account.

Your maintenance level of calories is the number of calories you require to maintain your weight right now. If there is no accurate calculator to do this, how do you figure out what this number is? You track what you're eating right now. Simple as that.

For one full week, you should track your weight and everything you ate, every day.

You want to be as specific as you can be. Record the amounts, the food itself, and the calories. You also want to weigh yourself every morning before you eat or drink and after you go to the bathroom.

Don't fudge the numbers, don't sneak unrecorded food, and don't try to be "good" just because you're keeping track. Just eat whatever you normally eat and keep track of it. While practicing flexible dieting, you're going to be tracking your food eventually, so you might as well get used to it now.

Add up all of your calories consumed and divide it by seven. This was your average daily caloric intake.

If you lost weight over this time, you're eating under your maintenance. If you gained, then you were eating over your maintenance. If you maintained, well, those are your maintenance calories. Every pound contains roughly 3500 calories. So, if you divide 3500 by the change in weight, you have the number of calories you were over or under your maintenance for the week.

FINDING MAINTENANCE CALORIES

1 ENDING WEIGHT - STARTING WEIGHT = WEIGHT CHANGE

2 (3500 X WEIGHT CHANGE) ÷ 7 = DEVIATION FROM YOUR MAINTENANCE

3 (ADD UP ALL 7 DAYS OF CALORIES) ÷ 7 = AVERAGE DAILY CALORIC INTAKE

4 AVERAGE DAILY CALORIC INTAKE ± / - DEVIATION FROM MAINTENANCE = MAINTENANCE CALORIES

If you lost weight over the week, you ADD the deviation from maintenance to your average daily caloric intake. If you gained weight, you SUBTRACT it from your average daily caloric intake.

This was a lot of numbers, so here the whole formula written out for you.

This is the most accurate way to find out where you currently are, calorically and metabolically speaking. This method is far more accurate than any calculator on the planet.

WHY CALORIES MATTER

When it comes down to it, weight loss and weight gain are both determined by caloric balance.[14] I think most of us understand the concept that when we eat more calories than we burn, we gain weight, and when we eat fewer calories than we burn, we lose weight. No matter how clean, whole, or unprocessed a food is, if you eat over your caloric maintenance, no matter the source, you will gain weight[15]. Calories in versus calories out are on the bottom line of any physique goal, so they do matter.

(Now it's more complex than it sounds on the surface because of the nuances of how many calories we're eating and absorbing and how many calories each person burns, but the bottom line is this statement is true no matter what.)

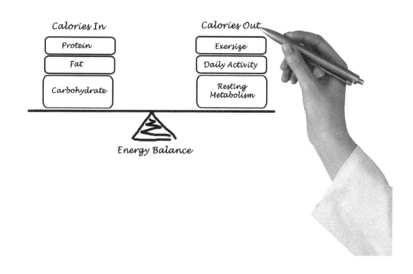

However, they are not *all* that matters. The type of macros your calories come from will determine what *kind* of tissue you gain or lose (in conjunction with your training of course). For example, you can lose 20 pounds by restricting calories alone, but without planning your macronutrients, and weight training appropriately, the weight lost is far more likely to be coming from muscle[16]. Conversely, you can definitely gain weight by eating a surplus of calories, but without a clue where they are coming from, you can easily gain more fat than you intended[15].

A WORD ABOUT METABOLISM

Most people think of their metabolism as an unchangeable trait, like their height or eye color.

"I have green eyes."

"I have a slow metabolism."

That's the way it is taught, and that is often the way it is portrayed in health and fitness publications. I am here to say that it is not so. Your metabolism changes. It is in no way static.

Your metabolism is actually quite good at adapting to new stimulus and can change dramatically in relatively short periods. There are some theories that you can even change your actual genetic set point over longer periods of time.[17]

Now, these changes can be good or bad depending on what you do (and of course "good" and "bad" are subject to the individual and that individual's goals), but the point is that it can change. So, just because you have found your caloric baseline for *now* doesn't mean that's what it will be forever. Your diet, your work environment, your sleeping patterns, your workouts, muscle gain, fat loss, and even your age can play big roles in how efficiently your metabolism burns energy.

You are not chained to your current metabolism for life.

DETERMINING YOUR GOALS

Setting your goals is a crucial, but often overlooked step in determining how you are going to set up your diet. Be realistic in your goal setting, and don't be afraid to ease your way into it by starting with "Maintenance Macros" and transitioning into "Cutting" or "Building" macros as you get used to the process.

Since you have determined the number of calories needed to maintain your weight, you now need to decide whether you want your weight to stay the same, go down, or go up, ideally by way of building muscle and/or shedding fat. As discussed above, you will need to eat more than your maintenance calories to build muscle, and less than your maintenance calories to shed fat.

"BUT I WANT TO BUILD MUSCLE AND BURN FAT!"

If I had a dollar for every time I heard this! And who can blame anyone? Don't we all want to build muscle and burn fat at the same time? But the sad fact is that it is very, very difficult (some would say impossible) for someone to do both simultaneously.

This isn't to say that it absolutely can't be done. It can be done, but usually at a very slow pace. The exceptions to this rule are:

- Beginners, untrained individuals, and people brand new to exercise.
- People using anabolic steroids.

- People with fantastic genetics.
- People returning to fitness after a year or more off.
- Young people, often still in puberty.

However, even these lucky folks will hit a sticking point eventually. At that point it is best to focus more on one goal: muscle building, or fat loss; bulking or cutting; growing or shrinking. And you don't have to be married to that goal forever. You can cycle through them in short or long bursts, or just work to where you want to be, and maintain from there.

MAINTENANCE OR BODY RE-COMPOSITION

If you are already a healthy weight that you're comfortable with and are just looking to tweak your body fat levels, but not necessarily drop or gain much weight, maintenance, or body re-composition is a good place to start. Also, if you are new to exercising, and/or have a significant amount of weight to lose, maintenance is a great place start. As you begin to exercise more frequently, the number of calories you burn will increase, thus creating a larger caloric deficit within this category.

Seasoned athletes can also do well in a maintenance stage for a long while, just tweaking things slowly as they go to enhance performance, without gaining or losing significant amounts of weight, or losing strength, speed or power.

MUSCLE BUILDING

If you are on the smaller or thinner side and are looking to add mass to your frame, you may choose to focus on building. Note that you will be eating *more* calories than your maintenance level in order to build tissue. The larger the surplus, the faster the gain will happen, but the more likely you are to also add some fat. The smaller the surplus, the more likely the tissue gained will be mostly muscle (with proper training), but it will be a slower process.

FAT LOSS

If you are looking to lose some fat or weight, but maintain your muscle, this is where you want to be. You will be eating *less* than your maintenance calories in order to create the caloric deficit needed to lose fat. The larger the deficit, the more likely you are to lose muscle tissue as well as fat. The smaller the deficit, the more likely you are to lose mostly fat, and while it takes longer, the results are also generally longer lasting. This fact assumes you are following a sound resistance-training program.

5 CALCULATING YOUR MACROS

This is really the foundation of the book, figuring out your own unique macros. It is important to remember though, that these are not absolute-100%-sure-fire-figures-for-the-rest-of-your-life macros. They are estimates, albeit thorough and well planned, they are starting ballpark figures. Each macro target has ranges, and you can feel free to experiment within those ranges to find what feels best for you and gets you the best results. But this is a great jumping off point.

CALORIES

Previously, we discussed how to determine your maintenance caloric level, and we also discussed various goals and what they mean. Hopefully, you have decided which direction you'd like to go and at this point, we can determine your starting calorie intake.

Maintenance / Body Re-Composition:

For maintenance and body re-composition goals, all you need to do is keep your calories the same and use this as your caloric number in the macro calculations below.

Muscle Building:

In a building phase, you need to decide how much you want to build and how fast. This will determine your caloric surplus. The more calories you add, the faster you will gain weight, and the higher the likelihood of fat gain. The fewer you add, the longer it will take to gain weight, but there is a lower likelihood of fat gain. I personally always like to err on the side of slower weight gain. This makes dieting a less painful process later, should you decide to eventually cut calories. This being said, to enter a building phase you can add anywhere from 200-600 calories to your maintenance calories. A 500-calorie surplus per day, in theory, should result in a 1 pound of weight gain per week. Gaining more than this (unless you are starting from a very thin or even underweight place), generally means that you are gaining fat as well as muscle.

Fat Loss:

Conversely, cutting calories means we will need to create a caloric deficit, and you need to determine how quickly you'd like to do this. The larger the deficit and the faster you lose weight, the more likely it is you will lose muscle. And the smaller the deficit, the slower you lose weight, but it is less likely to be muscle and more likely to be fat loss. In addition to that, I would like to add that slower weight loss is typically more maintainable and is longer lasting than crash dieting. From your maintenance calories, you can subtract anywhere from 200-800 calories per day to enter a fat loss phase. If you are losing more than 1-2 pounds per week, you are almost certainly losing some muscle.

For our example, let's use a 180-pound person (Let's call him Jack), with a maintenance level of calories that is 2300. He wants to enter a fat loss phase at a moderate pace. His calorie calculation would be:

SETTING JACK'S CALORIES

$$2400 - 400 = 2000 \text{ CALORIES}$$

Caloric Maintenance	Size of deficit	Daily Calories while in Fat Loss Phase

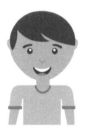

***Set your caloric deficit anywhere from 200-800 calories fewer than your caloric maintenance. A steeper deficit may mean more muscle loss and will be harder to adhere to. Do not go below 1300 for women and 1800 for men without professional guidance.

PROTEIN

Protein is the first macronutrient you should calculate. To determine your protein requirements, you will need to estimate your body fat percentage. It doesn't need to be exact, as almost no method will give you a perfectly accurate measurement, but be honest with yourself. A few ways you could go about finding your rough body fat calculations are

- Going to a nearby gym and seeing if a trainer can measure you with calipers
- Ordering a pair of calipers online and learning how to measure yourself.
- Getting a "dunk test" or hydrostatic weighing.
- Getting a Dexa Scan (This is the most accurate method, but also quite expensive)

I don't recommend hand held scales or bio-impedance body fat scales because they are usually so far off that it isn't even worth using them as a guide.

If you have *no* idea where to start, the following chart can be a good starting place, although it will obviously not be perfect since everyone stores fat differently, and everyone has a different amount of muscle mass. Again, it doesn't have to be exact, but typically speaking, our body fat is usually higher than we think, so bear that in mind.

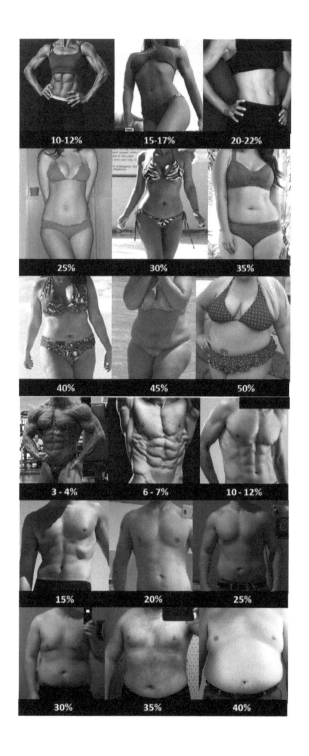

Once you have your rough body fat percentage, multiply it by your weight in pounds. Then subtract your answer from your weight. What you are left with is your lean body mass (LBM), or the fat free mass in your body. This is skeletal muscle, bone, connective tissue, and organs.

JACK'S LEAN BODY MASS

Jack estimates he is at 20% body fat.

180 X .20 = 36 LB BODY FAT
Body   % body   Pounds of Body Fat
Weight   fat

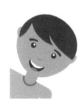

180 - 36 = 144 LB LEAN
Body   Pounds   **BODY MASS**
Weight   of fat

The amount of protein you require is based on your lean body mass. You should be aiming to get anywhere from .8-1.2g of protein per pound of lean body mass, depending on your goals.[7] This is a fairly large range, and where you decide to fall in the range can be determined by a few guidelines.

People in a building phase and younger people in general can stay on the lower end, about .8-1g/ pound LBM. Those in a fat loss phase and older people (50+) should stick to the higher end around 1-1.2 g per pound of LBM.[7] If you are in a maintenance phase, you can play around within the range to find what suits you best.

Let's take Jack, who is going into a fat loss phase. His calculation would look something like this:

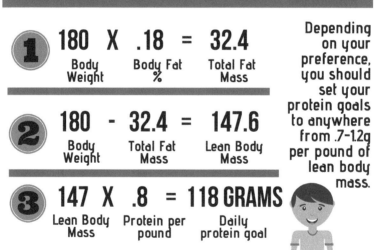

SETTING JACK'S PROTEIN TARGET

1 $180 \times .18 = 32.4$
Body Weight · Body Fat % · Total Fat Mass

2 $180 - 32.4 = 147.6$
Body Weight · Total Fat Mass · Lean Body Mass

3 $147 \times .8 = 118\ GRAMS$
Lean Body Mass · Protein per pound · Daily protein goal

Depending on your preference, you should set your protein goals to anywhere from .7-1.2g per pound of lean body mass.

Pro Tip: Many people can stop right here! If you're brand new to tracking your food and are already feeling overwhelmed by all of these numbers, you can focus on these two numbers to start: your calories, and your protein.

If you can hit these two numbers regularly, you are in a great place, and you will likely see results from this alone. As you become more confident in the process of tracking and reaching your protein goals, then you can start calculating your carbs and fats and trying to reach those numbers as well. But there is no need to rush things. You are more likely to succeed if you take it one manageable step at a time rather than ambushing yourself with a dozen new meticulous goals.

FAT

Fat should be the second macronutrient to calculate, just for simplicity's sake. Determining your fat requirements will be dependent on your preferences. Which do you prefer: carbs or fats? Because the more fat you have, the fewer carbohydrates you will get and vice versa.

When I ask which you prefer, what I mean is which do you find makes you feel the most satisfied? Which gives you better workouts? Better sleep? Better focus in your daily life? These are important questions to ask if you've never thought about it before, but once you've been practicing flexible dieting for a little while, you will start to figure out the answers for yourself.

If you're scratching your head over this one, I will say that you can safely fall anywhere in the range of having 20-40% of your calories coming from fat. For hormonal health reasons, and the absorption of fat-soluble vitamins, I would not recommend going below 30g fat for women and 40g for men.[18]

Jack likes fat, but he's not crazy about it. He may calculate in the middle of the range, like so:

SETTING JACK'S FAT TARGET

$$2000 \times .30 = 600 \text{ CALS}$$

Daily Calories   % cals from fat   calories from fat

$$600 \div 9 = 67 \text{ GRAMS}$$

calories from fat   cals per gram fat   daily fat target

Depending on your preference, fat can make up 20-40% of your daily calories, but do not go below 30g for women and 40g for men.

CARBOHYDRATES

The most manipulated macro will almost always be carbs. Carbs can be manipulated in many ways (some of which we will get to later) to stimulate fat-loss, to promote muscle growth, to give you immediate energy when needed, to boost hormone levels, and to give you killer workouts.

So, there's a lot we can do with carbs. For our purposes at this point, we are going to fill our remaining calories with carbs. How we do this will require the most math you will need to do in this whole book. (It's not that bad though, I promise.)

You take the number of calories you're going to be eating and subtract the calories from protein (by multiplying the grams by 4, which is the number of calories per gram of protein). Then also subtract the calories from fat (by multiplying the grams by 9, which is the number of calories per gram of fat). What you are left with is the number of calories that will be coming from carbohydrates.

Divide this number by 4 (the number of calories per gram of carbohydrates) and you have your carbohydrate goal for the day. In simpler terms:

(Protein x 4) + (Fat x 9) = Calories from protein and fat

Total calories – Protein and Fat calories = Carb calories

Carb calories ÷ 4 = Carbohydrate grams

If that was confusing, here's Jack to show us how it's done.

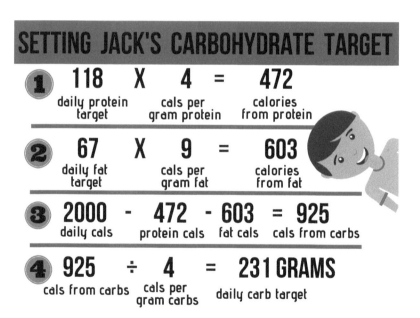

SETTING JACK'S CARBOHYDRATE TARGET

1 118 X 4 = 472
daily protein target | cals per gram protein | calories from protein

2 67 X 9 = 603
daily fat target | cals per gram fat | calories from fat

3 2000 - 472 - 603 = 925
daily cals | protein cals | fat cals | cals from carbs

4 925 ÷ 4 = 231 GRAMS
cals from carbs | cals per gram carbs | daily carb target

FIBER

I'm not going to discuss this one too much because I'm not concerned that any vegan won't get enough fiber. Just to cover my bases however, have 14g of fiber per 1000 calories as a *minimum*. For Jack who is consuming 2000 calories per day, this would be 28g.

You should establish an upper limit for yourself as well, and this will vary from person to person, so pay attention to your body's reactions. As a general guideline though, I like to keep my cap at no more than 30g per 1000 calories. For Joe, this would be 60g.

The most important thing about fiber is to be fairly consistent with how much you have every day. Try to eat in about a 10g range on most days.

And there we have established the baseline macros for your goals! Now, what do we do with these three numbers?

6 TRACKING, COUNTING AND LOGGING YOUR FOOD

Tracking your food is not fun. Whew, glad I got that out of the way.

There's nothing glamorous about it. It's tedious, and it gets old fast. I'd be lying if I told you otherwise. But, and this is a big but, it is *crucial* to track your food with flexible dieting, especially while you are learning how to do it. Tracking your food is non-negotiable.

If you've never tracked your eating habits before (but you should have to find your maintenance calories!), this could be a big eye opener for you. Many people do not even realize how much they have been over-eating, or under-eating. Most people have no idea what their food is actually comprised of, so tracking your food for long enough can teach you a lot about yourself both physically and mentally.

You will need to regularly use a food scale, at least until you get accustomed to what food serving sizes look like. This will take a while. You can test yourself along the way by guessing and then putting a portion on the scale to see how close you are. (See? Just turn it into a game!).

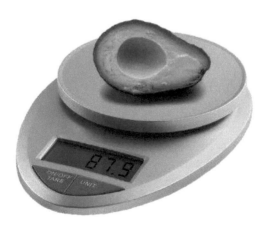

You'll be shocked at how accurately you can guess with enough practice. You can use measuring cups for liquids, but for solid foods, the scale is much more accurate than measuring cups. Measuring cups can vary when measuring food, depending on whether it's a level scoop, or how much the food has settled in a package, or even how the food is chopped. The scale, however, does not lie. Case in point: Weigh out 16 g of peanut butter on the scale. Then, measure a tablespoon of peanut butter in a measuring spoon and weigh *that*. I bet you dollars to donuts that the one in the measuring spoon weighs more.

There are four key points to being successful with food tracking: consistency, recording *honestly*, and having a plan daily.

Being consistent with your food tracking is so, so, so important in achieving the results you're going for, especially in the beginning. You should be tracking everything you eat for a couple of reasons. Every time you weigh and log something, it is practice, and you will eventually get better at it and it will become second nature, but like anything else, you have to put in the effort until you really "get it." Secondly, tracking everything helps you to hold yourself accountable. You're far less likely to sit on the couch and plow through a bag of chips if you know you're going to have to record it later.

Food logging will be a wasted effort if you're not being honest about what you're eating. You can't play the "if I didn't log it, it didn't happen" game and expect to get the results you want. Snacking while you're cooking, the beer you had out with your pals, and that heap of BBQ Sauce you put on your tofu----yeah, that all counts, so you should track it.

Also, do you know what five ounces of tofu looks like? Most people don't, and that makes sense; why would they? But guessing how much something weighs by eyeballing it can throw you way off your whole day's goals, especially if you do it regularly. That could easily set you back a week. Accuracy is crucial, so use your scale whenever you can until you're an estimating pro.

MY FITNESS PAL

The way you decide to track your food is up to you. You can use an app, pen and paper, make an excel spreadsheet, or keep a running note on your phone. But I can't speak highly enough about the My Fitness Pal (MFP) app, which you can download for free to any smartphone, or use on a desktop.

Disclaimer: Don't EVER, under any circumstances, use the preset macronutrient or caloric "suggestions" that MFP gives you after you punch in your body weight, age, goals, etc. They're garbage. Utter garbage. More on this later . . .

My Fitness Pal has an incredible amount of versatility and once you've logged a few days of food, it gets easier and easier. The food database alone makes it worthwhile; it contains nearly everything. I can count the number of times on one hand that it hasn't had a food that I was looking for in its database, *including* things like meals from certain restaurants, like Veggie Grill or TGIFridays.

There are many ways to enter foods, depending on how precise you want to be. You can enter foods based on "serving sizes" as suggested on the labels or you can enter foods in units such as "medium apple". Because I like to be as precise as possible, I like to enter any food that doesn't come out of a package in grams, which is the most accurate method. The easiest way to find food in grams is to just search for the food with the word "grams" after it. For example, if I want to find cooked brown rice in grams, I would type "cooked brown rice grams" into the search bar.

You can add your own recipes, you can scan barcodes of pre-packaged foods, you can save meals that you frequently have, and you can copy meals from previous days. It's very easy on the user, and I'm all about user-friendly things that make my life easier.

HAVING A PLAN OF ATTACK

Although flexible dieting is about being, well, flexible, having at least a loose plan is going to be incredibly helpful to your success.

Whether you want to plan your food a day in advance or a full week in advance, flexible dieting still allows you the freedom to work in the foods that you enjoy. As you become more skilled at these methods, you will be able to improvise through the day more frequently. Trying to wing it from the get-go, however, is a recipe for failure when you're learning. Walk before you run, my friend.

I personally like to plan my daily meals in the morning, but many people like to do it the night before. I pretty much always eat the same thing for breakfast (creature of habit), and then I take about 5 minutes to plan the rest of my day. This way, I have a plan, and if it changes a little bit, it's easy to manipulate a few grams here and there, but overall, I know what I'm going to do.

Some days I *do* wing it, but I've also been doing this for years. In the beginning, have a plan that works for you and that you feel confident about and branch out from there as you become more comfortable.

Putting your food into MFP a day, or even a week in advance is also great because, once it's logged, you're much more likely to eat it. And also, as you get used to it, buying groceries becomes both more fun than eating a strict meal plan, and also allows you to not buy a bunch of extras, because you already have a rough idea of what you're going to eat.

WHY IS MY FITNESS PAL TELLING ME TO EAT 1200 CALORIES?

For all of the reasons that I love My Fitness Pal, I absolutely *loathe* its caloric calculations. It uses a basic calorie calculator from the data that you enter when you sign up for an account. As discussed earlier in the book, standard calorie calculators are wildly inaccurate, but by telling you a number of calories you should eat (and not explaining how they came to that number) they make you think, "I need to eat X calories to hit my goals." As a society, we like to focus on numbers; we like concrete goals and MFP plays on that by creating one for you, but it is usually horribly off, and can cause more harm than good.

When you sign up for a My Fitness Pal account, the program prompts you with several questions about your current weight and your goals. It then uses a basic calculator to calculate your "maintenance" calories—see, that is in quotes because it always wrong. And any woman who has ever selected the goal of losing "2 pounds per week" then automatically has 1000 calories slashed from that maintenance number (something I do *not* generally recommend), which is usually well under 1200. *But,* since the general consensus is that anything under 1200 is unhealthy and something not able to be maintained, it defaults to 1200 so as not to drop dangerously low. And *that,* my friends, is how the magical 1200 number came to be. Mystery solved. It's not a magic number. It's a computer programming error that has turned into a widespread phenomenon resulting in thousands of women who severely under-eat.

HOW TO SET YOUR CUSTOM MACRO GOALS

In my original writing of this book, there was a nifty hack to set your macros to custom numbers in My Fitness Pal. Shortly after the release of the book, MFP grew wise to this hack and started charging a premium for this feature.

The easiest way to set your macros to custom numbers is to pay for the premium version. As of the writing of this, it is $10 a month or $50 for the year. I have paid the yearly subscription since day 1, and I love it. You have access to many exclusive features, and also, there are no ads.

However, I understand not everyone wants to pay for an ongoing macro tracker so I will give you a tip on how to set it as close as possible.

From your home page in your app, click the "…" in the lower right-hand corner. From here, click "Goals", then click "Calories, Carbs, Protein and Fat Goals". From here you can change things.

First, set your calories to the caloric goal we calculated in the last chapter. Next you can set the fat goal to the percentage you chose from the last chapter as well (20-40%). After this, you have to play with the toggles a bit on the protein and carbs to get as close as possible to your target numbers. It may not be perfect, but that is ok! Just get as close as you can, click the checkmark, and go back to your home screen.

WHY IS MY CALORIE TOTAL ALWAYS WRONG?

This is a part that confuses and frustrates a lot of people: your calories are going to be wrong more often than not by the end of the day. Unless you're following the protein + calories only method listed in the previous chapter, don't even look at the calories on My

Fitness Pal from here on out. Just pay attention to protein, carbs, fat and fiber. "But Dani, I thought that the number of calories we need to hit was the basis of all of this planning?! Now you're saying to ignore that?!" Well, yes and no.

Calories *do* matter, and they *are* the basis for all our calculations. They are **the** most important thing for weight loss or gain. But remember, each gram of protein and carbs have 4 calories, and each gram of fat has 9 calories, so if you are hitting your macros, then you *are* hitting your calories!

But they will almost never add up to what you set them to, and it will infuriate you.

Why does this happen? In the USA (and it varies from country to country), food companies are allowed to skew the numbers on their nutrition labels by excluding fiber calories.[19] What's worse is that only some companies actually do this, so it is inconsistent.

If you've hit your macros at the end of the day, but your calories are way off, don't sweat it. You're right and they are wrong—it makes no sense.

For example, let's take a look at this label. This is Joseph's Flax, Oat Bran and Whole Wheat Pita—one of my favorites.

Joseph's Middle East Bakery
Reduced Carb/Flax, Oat Bran & Whole Wheat Pita
Bread
6 pack

Nutrition Facts

Serving Size: 1 Pita (37g/1.33oz)
Servings Per Container: 6

	Amount Per Serving	% Daily Value*
Total Calories	60	
Calories From Fat	20	
Total Fat	2 g	3%
Saturated Fat	0 g	0%
Trans Fat	0 g	
Cholesterol	0 mg	0%
Sodium	300 mg	13%
Total Carbohydrates	8 g	3%
Dietary Fiber	4 g	16%
Sugars	0 g	
⊞ Show Net Carbs		
Protein	6 g	

8g carbs   x 4 = 32 calories from carbs
6g protein   x 4 = 24 calories from protein
2g fat   x 9 = 18 calories from fat
32 + 24 + 18 = 74 Total Calories

But the label says 60 calories. Hmmmm…. Now let's subtract the fiber calories and take a look.

4g fiber   x 4 = 16 calories
74 calories   - 16 fiber calories = 58 calories.

So, you can see they subtracted the fiber calories and rounded to 60 calories. And there are many, many companies that do this. The point here is, your calories will never line up exactly to what you want them to in MFP, but as long as you're hitting your macros, you're good.

SHOULD I TRACK FRUITS AND VEGGIES?

Fruits and vegetables should be tracked. While you don't need to get super obsessed with weighing every piece of lettuce you have, the stricter your goal is, the more closely you need to track.

But, as vegans, a cup of broccoli is more like a garnish to us (can you believe that's actually a serving to a lot of people?), and we think nothing of wiping out a pound at a time, which can easily add up to 150-200 calories. Obviously, these are super nutrient dense foods, and should make up a large part of your diet. But track them like anything else.

SHOULD I SUBTRACT FIBER OR TRACK NET CARBS?

No, you should not subtract fiber. Although fiber is not digested in the same way that other carbohydrates are, a portion of them are broken down into fatty acids, and you do absorb calories from them.[20] Do not worry about net carbs, and do not subtract fiber from your carbohydrate count. Count them all.

WHAT ABOUT SODIUM AND SUGAR?

Many people have questions about sodium and sugar when they begin tracking their food. Athletes require sodium and carbohydrates, many of which are sugar, are the body's first fuel source.

If you are sodium sensitive or have high blood pressure problems, watch your sodium and keep it where your doctor has recommended. I am not in the business of overriding doctor's orders. But if you don't have issues with sodium and you're regularly exercising and breaking a sweat, sodium is important to keep your electrolytes in balance.[21] Your body is regulating your electrolyte and water levels minute to minute, so as long as you keep your sodium fairly consistent day to day, you shouldn't have issues with bloat or water retention, even if your sodium is on the higher side.

As far as sugar goes, I have found that if you are getting enough fiber and hitting your other macros, it is not easy to get too much sugar. As a general rule of thumb, I aim to have my total sugar (including natural sugars) be less than double my fiber. This isn't a hard and fast rule and endurance athletes will break this rule often to get in their necessary carbs and that is ok.

Obviously certain medical conditions, like diabetes, should be treated differently as explained by your doctor. But for someone without those conditions, I wouldn't worry about sugar much as long as you get enough fiber and stay within your carbohydrate goal.

SHOULD I LOG MY EXERCISE?

No. Do not log your exercise in My Fitness Pal. When you log your exercise in MFP, it automatically changes your caloric and macro goals for the day. Since we took into account your current maintenance level of calories, *including* your current workouts, you should not be logging exercise in MFP. If you want to keep track of your exercise, which I always recommend, you can use your phone's notepad, or a fantastic app called Strong.

DO I EAT BACK CALORIES I BURN?

Another big question people have, particularly those who use MFP regularly is, "Should I eat back the calories I burn during exercise?" No. You have already calculated your goals based on your current lifestyle, including your training, so you don't need to "eat back" exercise calories, because they are already accounted for. Trying to do so often gets far too complicated, and most people (and cardio machines, and calculators) largely overestimate how many calories are actually burned during exercise.

The exception to this is an out of the ordinary physical event, like a long race or an all-day hike. In this case, I would suggest looking at it on a case-by-case basis and adding calories accordingly.

7   THE THREE-TIERED APROACH TO TRACKING

In this book, we are specifically talking about flexible dieting via tracking all of your macro-nutrients. But there are other ways of tracking that can be very effective as well and I want to touch upon those for a moment.

You see, after years of teaching this methodology, which I still stand firmly behind, I have found that some people can get *very* rigid about their macronutrients, to the point that there is nothing flexible about it.

Aside from this having mental implications of stress on the individual, it also leads them back down this path of black and white thinking which is precisely what flexible dieting aims to avoid. This often manifests when someone misses one macro target and feels like they've blown the whole day and completely abandons the goal. This is absolutely not how to go about it.

We will all have occasional days where, for whatever reason, we simply cannot hit our macros. Whether it's travel, or a party, or simply that we overslept and messed up our meal schedule – these days will happen, and **it doesn't have to stop you from reaching your goals!**

In order to properly explain this, we need to dive into the nutritional hierarchy of how any physique change (weight gain, weight loss, muscle building, fat loss, etc.) works. Examine this graphic.

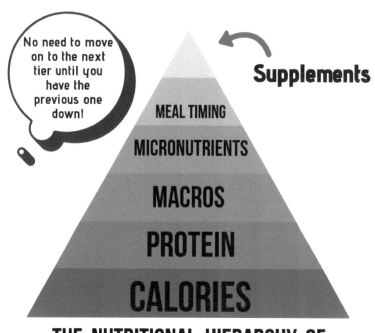

THE NUTRITIONAL HIERARCHY OF IMPORTANCE FOR FAT LOSS

Much like a real pyramid, no layer can stand without the layer beneath it solidly supporting it. Nutrition is the same way. In order to achieve your physique goals, you MUST have the lower parts of the pyramid in place.

As you can see, the basis of everything, as discussed in previous chapters, are calories. To gain or lose weight, your calories must be appropriate. Where I often see missteps here is if someone realizes they're going to miss their protein target, but because they've already gone over their carbs and/or fats, trying to reach the protein goal now would put them way over their calorie goal. **THAT** would thwart progress.

Above that, we see protein is the most important macronutrient **for physique change.**

Above that is where this book is largely based: on all three macronutrients.

Above that we have micronutrients, which are **incredibly** important for overall health, but less of a priority in physique change.

Above that we have some nuances of meal timing and eventually supplements which make the tiniest difference, but that people often jump to first!

So, to try and focus on meal timing when you continually miss your caloric goal makes no sense and you'd be much better served by just trying to achieve the caloric goal daily.

Now to explain the tier system and how you can best implement it.

GOOD:

- Hit your calorie goal within a 100-calorie range.

BETTER:

- Hit your calorie goal within a 100-calorie range.
- Hit your protein goal within a 20-gram range.

BEST:

- Hit your calorie goal within a 100-calorie range.
- Hit your protein and carbohydrate goal within a 20-gram range.
- Hit your fat goal within a 10-gram range.

BONUS PERFECT:

- Hit your calorie goal within a 100-calorie range.
- Hit your protein and carbohydrate goal within a 20-gram range.
- Hit your fat goal within a 10-gram range.

- Spread your protein out fairly evenly in 3-6 meals per day.
- Eat 20-30% of your carbohydrates both before and after your workouts.
- Keep your pre and post workout meals low in fat.

Now, you should always aim for the highest tier that you confidently can in order to make the best progress possible. But I would say 90% of people can make **outstanding** progress at the "Better" tier. And even the "Good" tier is wonderful for people who have over 30 pounds to lose. So, if you need to spend most of your time operating at one of these tiers – that is more than ok!

Some incidents when you might want to drop down a tier or two are:

- When you've accidentally gone over a macro by mid-day.
- When you know you have a big social engagement coming up,
- On vacation

- When someone surprises you with lunch or dinner out or cooks you a meal.
- When you're feeling burnt out on tracking so closely.
- When you're traveling and don't have access to your usual foods.
- When you're sick.

You wouldn't go slash all four tires if you got one flat. Do not sabotage your diet if you're off on one thing. Please use these tiers **guilt free** whenever you need to in order to retain the true sense of flexible dieting sustainably.

8 MEAL TIMING

For decades now, we have been beat over the head with the importance of eating 6 small meals a day to "speed up the metabolism" and "trick the body into burning more fat."

First of all, you're not going to trick your body into doing anything. It is much smarter than you or I. But more importantly, as more scientific studies are released, all of this talk about 6 small meals every 2-3 hours is turning out to be untrue.[24]

However, this doesn't mean that the importance of all meal timing should be thrown out the window. There are some basic components of meal timing that can be used by anyone. For more advanced athletes and those who are now confident in their ability to hit their macros regularly, fine-tuning meal timing can be very beneficial to athletic performance.

HOW MANY MEALS SHOULD I HAVE?

The most important factor in deciding how many meals you should eat per day is the answer to the question: What works for your lifestyle?

If you're on the road all day and find it easier to graze and have 6 small meals a day, by all means, go for it! But if you prefer to have sit-down dinners with your family, maybe you would prefer three square meals, and that is okay, too.

People with muscle building goals may find it easier to eat smaller meals more frequently to avoid bloating and gas from very large meals. Likewise, people cutting calories can often benefit from larger, but more infrequent meals because it actually allows the dieter to feel full and satisfied while in a caloric deficit.

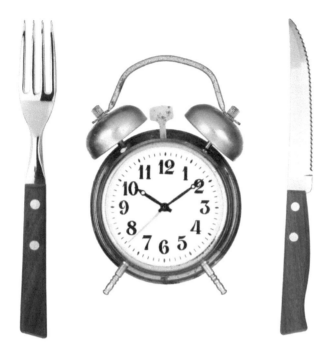

A good general recommendation for number of meals is 3-6. Research suggests that we can stimulate muscle protein synthesis anywhere from 3-6 times per day. This is very important for both building and maintaining muscle and it's something that we should try to stay within as much as we can.

When we eat protein in the right amounts, we stimulate muscle protein synthesis (MPS, the process of muscle repair and rebuilding).[25] We can only stimulate MPS 3-5 times a day, so I like to divide my protein intake evenly over that many meals to capitalize on this.[26]

It's for this reason that I do not recommend one-meal-a-day, sometimes called OMAD. OMAD is a style of intermittent fasting where, you guessed it, you only have one meal a day and fast for the rest of the day. While I do think that Intermittent fasting can be helpful when cutting as it narrows your eating window, allowing you to feel more satisfied during that time frame, I think that is where the intermittent fasting's benefits mostly end. With just one feeding per day, you leave 2-4 episodes of muscle protein synthesis - muscle building - on the table and you're much more likely to burn through muscle tissue when fasting.

EATING FOR PERFORMANCE. PRE & POST WORKOUT MEALS.

You can stop organizing your meal timing right here and make great progress. But let's say you want to take it a step farther than this. How could you set up your meal timing to optimize your performance? The theories of beneficial meal timing mostly revolve around muscle protein synthesis and glycogen storage for better workouts.

Protein: Once you've decided how many meals you plan to have, divide your protein goal by that number and try to eat roughly that much protein at each meal. Aside from the muscle repairing benefits, trying to eat all of (or most of) your protein in one sitting, is almost guaranteed to bring some digestive discomfort, if you know what I mean. Athlete or not, I recommend splitting up protein fairly evenly between however many meals you plan to have. This is the same during building, fat loss, and maintenance phases.

Carbohydrates: The next step is to focus on carbohydrates. If you work out hard or regularly and you want to maximize your workouts, it is a good idea to concentrate a large portion of your carbohydrates around your workouts.[27] I like to have 40-60% of my daily carbs around my workouts (20-30% both before and after), and then spread the rest through the day however I'd like.

Fat: When looking at dietary fat, more important than *when* to have fat, is *when not* to have fat, which is around your workouts. Your pre- and post-workout meals should each be low in fat, no more than 10% of your daily fat. The reason for this is that fat slows down the digestion of the rest of your meal.[28] Before and after your workouts, you want that energy to be taken in as quickly as possible. The rest of the day, however, spread your fats out however you'd like, especially during the time of day when you are usually the hungriest, as fats are incredibly satiating.

EARLY RISERS

If you are one of those crazy people who wake up at the crack of dawn to work out, you're probably thinking that it would be impossible to get down that much protein and carbohydrate at 5 am. And honestly, you'd probably throw up during your burpees if you tried.

To these people, I suggest trying to eat a meal about half this size immediately upon waking, even though it is not ideal, it is better than nothing. Perhaps make a protein shake with a banana the night before and put it in the fridge so it's ready when you wake up.

Alternatively, the night before your workout, you can have 25-30% of your carbs with your last meal of the night, so that it keeps your glycogen stores full until morning, when you'll train fasted, and have your post workout meal as detailed above afterwards. It's not ideal, but it's still a good option for this specific scenario.

How close to training you have your pre- and post-workout meals depends upon what your stomach can handle. If you eat too much, or eat too soon before your training, you may throw up or get queasy because all of the energy your body would be using to digest your food is now being sent away from the stomach and to the muscles. This is not good.

I find that anywhere from 30 minutes to 2 hours before I go work out is a good time frame for my pre-workout meal. I try to eat my post-workout meal as soon as I get home, although anything up to about two hours is ok. I'm usually hungry right after training, as I imagine most people are.

9 PUTTING IT ALL TOGETHER

In this section we will be taking everything we have learned so far and actually putting it all into practice in your first actionable meal plan that you can get started on right away!

WHAT DO I EAT TO HIT THESE NUMBERS?

Whatever you want! Isn't that cool!? But truthfully, it will take a while to fully get the hang of what foods work to hit these numbers by the end of the day. One of the easiest things you can do for yourself is to make a list of foods you like that are high in either protein, carbohydrate, or fat. This simple reference will be so helpful when it comes time to put together your meal plan.

The number one issue that vegans have with flexible dieting, or IIFYM, is that they do not know how to hit their protein goals without going way over on carbs or fat or both. This can be very tricky, because unlike our omnivorous counterparts, basically all of our main protein sources contain trace amounts of carbs or fat, and often more than just trace amounts.

Non-vegans often think of foods as "a protein", "a carb" or "a fat" food. As vegans, we've waved goodbye to this kind of thinking long ago, because we know that there is protein in just about everything, right? Well, now it's about putting this train of thought to good use.

Basically, every food gets a certain percentage of its calories from each macro type: protein, carbs and fat. Let's take for example peanuts, which many of us have long thought of as a great source of protein.

Peanuts get 14% of their calories from protein, 15% of their calories from carbs, and

71% percent of their calories from fat! So, if anything, the last thing that peanuts are is "a protein food." This doesn't mean that peanuts don't supply protein, but you will see that they quickly add up the fat grams as well.

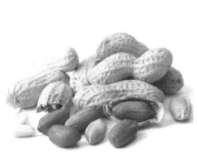
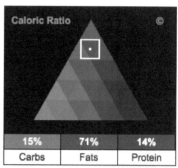

Now, let's take a look at black beans, another food that vegans commonly refer to as "protein." Black beans get 22% of their calories from protein (more than peanuts!), 3% of their calories from fat, and 75% percent of their calories from carbs. This is really more carbohydrates than anything else, even though it also has protein, which shouldn't be discounted.

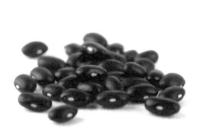
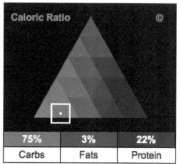

I call foods like these "protein extras." They are clearly more of a fat or carb than a protein, but don't discount the protein that is *does* have and that will go towards your protein total as well.

There are many high protein vegan foods that are lower in the other macronutrients such as tofu, seitan, certain brands of tempeh, mock meats (not all though, check the labels), plant-based protein powders, black bean pasta by Explore Asian, and on and on. You just have to know where to look.

In the Venn diagram following, I have illustrated plenty of vegan foods that fall into various categories. This is not an exhaustive list, and it changes all the time as companies come out with new products or reformulate, but it contains many, many vegan foods to help you hit your numbers. For example, if you are realizing that you are lacking in protein and carbs, you could either pick something that is higher in protein and carbs and lower in fat (like beans), or eat a smaller amount of a mostly protein food and a mostly carb food (like protein powder and a banana).

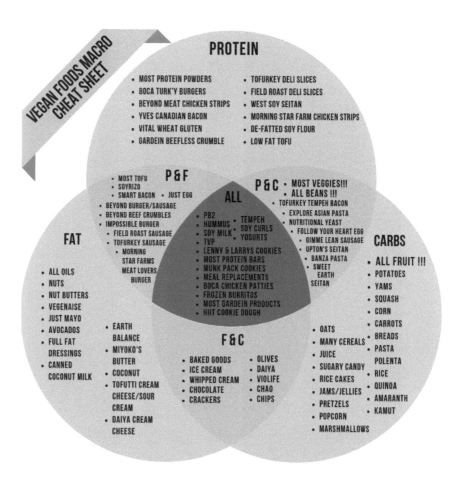

VEGAN FOODS MACRO CHEAT SHEET

PROTEIN

- MOST PROTEIN POWDERS
- BOCA TURK'Y BURGERS
- BEYOND MEAT CHICKEN STRIPS
- YVES CANADIAN BACON
- VITAL WHEAT GLUTEN
- GARDEIN BEEFLESS CRUMBLE

- TOFURKEY DELI SLICES
- FIELD ROAST DELI SLICES
- WEST SOY SEITAN
- MORNING STAR FARM CHICKEN STRIPS
- DE-FATTED SOY FLOUR
- LOW FAT TOFU

P&F
- MOST TOFU
- SOYRIZO
- SMART BACON • JUST EGG
- BEYOND BURGER/SAUSAGE
- BEYOND BEEF CRUMBLES
- IMPOSSIBLE BURGER
- FIELD ROAST SAUSAGE
- TOFURKEY SAUSAGE
- MORNING
  STAR FARMS
  MEAT LOVERS
  BURGER

ALL
- PB2
- HUMMUS • TEMPEH
- SOY MILK • SOY CURLS
- TVP • YOGURTS
- LENNY & LARRYS COOKIES
- MOST PROTEIN BARS
- MUNK PACK COOKIES
- MEAL REPLACEMENTS
- BOCA CHICKEN PATTIES
- FROZEN BURRITOS
- MOST GARDEIN PRODUCTS
- HIIT COOKIE DOUGH

P&C
- MOST VEGGIES!!!
- ALL BEANS !!!
- TOFURKEY TEMPEH BACON
- EXPLORE ASIAN PASTA
- NUTRITIONAL YEAST
- FOLLOW YOUR HEART EGG
- GIMME LEAN SAUSAGE
- UPTON'S SEITAN
- BANZA PASTA
- SWEET
  EARTH
  SEITAN

FAT

- ALL OILS
- NUTS
- NUT BUTTERS
- VEGENAISE
- JUST MAYO
- AVOCADOS
- FULL FAT
  DRESSINGS
- CANNED
  COCONUT MILK

- EARTH
  BALANCE
- MIYOKO'S
  BUTTER
- COCONUT
- TOFUTTI CREAM
  CHEESE/SOUR
  CREAM
- DAIYA CREAM
  CHEESE

F&C
- BAKED GOODS
- ICE CREAM
- WHIPPED CREAM
- CHOCOLATE
- CRACKERS

- OLIVES
- DAIYA
- VIOLIFE
- CHAO
- CHIPS

CARBS

- ALL FRUIT !!!
- POTATOES
- YAMS
- SQUASH
- CORN
- CARROTS
- OATS
- MANY CEREALS
- JUICE
- SUGARY CANDY
- RICE CAKES
- JAMS/JELLIES
- PRETZELS
- POPCORN
- MARSHMALLOWS
- BREADS
- PASTA
- POLENTA
- RICE
- QUINOA
- AMARANTH
- KAMUT

Many people think that to practice flexible dieting as a vegan you *have* to drink protein shakes. You don't! Even though I own VeganProteins.com, and sold vegan protein powders for nearly a decade, I personally rarely drink them, simply because I prefer food!

Food keeps me fuller for longer than a protein shake. Protein shakes do have their place and can definitely be more convenient when you're on the road, unprepared, or don't feel like eating. They also tend to be an optimal choice post workout because they are designed to have a great amino acid profile. But unless you're both soy free and gluten free (which you have no need to be if you don't have an allergy), you don't need to rely heavily on protein shakes.

I consume plenty of seitan, tofu, and mock meats. Actually, I rely more on mock-meat type foods as my calories get lower when I am cutting calories, simply because they are usually lower in fat and carbs than tofu and tempeh.

Since originally writing this book, I have received a lot of pushback on my love of mock meats. Please do not get me wrong, you can absolutely hit your macros without them, and you're welcome to! That's the beauty of flexible dieting. But mock meats are not as mysterious and processed (some are, but not all!) as they may seem. Many mock meats, seitan and even tofu can be made from scratch in your own kitchen from relatively simple ingredients.

If you've never taken a look, check out our Vegan Proteins YouTube channel to see dozens of recipe videos for making high protein vegan foods!

PRO TIP: Vegans have been told for a long time that too much protein is bad for us. There have been very few studies done on higher amounts of plant proteins, but what has been found thus far is that plant proteins don't have the same effect as animal proteins.[22] Many believe that too much protein is bad for the kidneys, but this is based on a study from 1983 that was later debunked. The findings showed that high protein diets (a fair amount higher than I have been recommending here) increased the amounts of blood filtered through kidneys (GFR, or globular filtration rate), but that it had no adverse or damaging effects in healthy kidneys.[23]

HOW TO CREATE YOUR INITIAL MEAL PLAN

Here we are going to put all of the pieces together and plan out a day's food in My Fitness Pal. You can then use this as a skeleton meal plan to get through the week and change it every week, a guide for your meal prep, or you can just stick to it like glue until you feel more comfortable!

First, make sure you set your custom macros as described in the previous chapter. If you do not have the premium My Fitness Pal, just get as close as you can with the percentages.

Next, set up your number of meals by clicking the "..." in the bottom corner, then clicking "Settings", then "Customize Meal Names". From here you can add or delete meals and give them the names you'd like (for example pre-workout, afternoon snack, etc.).

Ok, now we are ready to start plugging in foods. A couple of pro tips!

- Log these for a day in the future so you don't mess up your current day's tracking.

- Also, if you turn your phone sideways, you can see the macros of every food as you log them.

- Tapping the blue bar above each meal changes the % to grams.

Using all of the information from the previous chapters, you know your protein should be roughly evenly divided between all of your meals. So, if your protein goal is 125g and you have planned for 5 meals, you know you need about 25g protein per meal.

For your first logging step, choose your main protein source for each meal and plug in your protein amount per meal. This could be tofu, seitan, protein powder, tempeh or veggie bacon. This will seem like a lot of food first, but don't worry. We're going to come back and edit.

Next, plug in your veggies! This is to make sure that you are getting plenty of veggies early in the planning stages rather than trying to sneak them in at the end.

Now you're remember how we need to have 20-40% of our carbohydrates both before and after our workouts? Now we will plug those in with carb-heavy foods of your choice. This could be toast, oatmeal, fruit, beans or smarties. Be sure to keep those pre and post workout meals low in fat.

Add your remaining carbs to the rest of your meals as you wish.

Turn your phone to the side and you will see that you are probably significantly over on your protein now, so go back and reduce the amount of protein foods to get back to your original goal.

It's at this point I would recommend going back in and adding your main fat sources: nuts, nut butter, seeds, avocado, vegan cheese, olives etc. Fill in the gaps.

From here, you have your meals mostly plugged in, it is now about going back and tweaking the amounts until you hit your targets! To see this in real time, check out this video.

10 THE DREADED PLATEAU

Although no one likes to think this is going to happen to them, at some point you will hit a plateau. Plateaus are a completely normal, albeit frustrating, part of reaching any physique goal. Learning how to recognize a true plateau and how to react to it is just as important as calculating and hitting your initial macros.

As has been mentioned before, your body is a crazy efficient and complex machine, and it will adapt to nearly anything you throw at it, including new macros, training protocol, etc. Things will need to be tweaked over time.

And sometimes, you have to go back to the drawing board and start all over in order to keep making progress. But not too soon . . .

One major problem that I encounter over and over again in the fitness community is that people change things up way too frequently. Whether it's a meal plan, a set of macros, or even a training routine, people are constantly bouncing around from program to program and wondering why they aren't getting the results they want. Your body needs time to adapt and change with a program before starting a new one and macros are no different.

When someone recalculates their macros too frequently, they are setting themselves up for failure because they don't stick with something long enough to learn what works for them and what does not.

On the flip side, some people want to stay married to their macros and never change them once they've been figured out. Unfortunately, for most people, one set of macros will not take them all the way to their goal, and that's okay and totally normal. You will hit plateaus, and at that point, you should start tweaking.

GIVE YOUR MACROS A CHANCE

You just spent a great deal of energy calculating your starting macros—stick with them! Try and hit these macros consistently for **at least four weeks** and see how they are working out for you and your goals.

Your macros will need to be adjusted as you make progress, but don't change them just for the sake of changing them. Change them because you need to, not because you're bored or anxious about if they are possibly not working.

Patience is a virtue and a very important one with any physical goals because these changes do not happen overnight.

YOU CAN'T MANAGE WHAT YOU DON'T MEASURE

A key component to gauging your progress is to actually gauge your progress! I can't stress enough the importance of progress photos and measurements. Set up a time when you take photos and measurements, whether that is weekly, bi-weekly or monthly is up to you, but be sure to make this a priority.

If your main goal is to be building muscle, you're looking for weight gain and increased size, and increased muscular development in the photos. This doesn't mean the muscles look more defined - not means they look bigger. You will also find that areas of the body where do not store much fat (calves, biceps) will increase over time.

If your main goal is fat loss, you are looking for weight loss and/or more muscular definition in your progress photos. You may also find that places you store more body fat (navel, hips, thighs) will be decreasing over time.

If your main goal is maintenance and body re-composition, you will need to rely heavily on photos because measurements may be all over the place. How are your clothes fitting? How is your gym performance? How do the photos compare month to month?

I actually recorded an entire Muscles by Brussels Radio podcast episode on the best ways to gauge your progress in episode #6, which you can listen to for free on iTunes, Spotify or Stitcher.

WHAT TO DO WHEN PROGRESS STALLS

If you are still making progress, even if it's slow, don't change anything! I cannot stress this enough: if it ain't broke, don't fix it. If after checking your progress, you've found that you have not made any changes in 4 weeks, you can adjust your carbs and fats up or down accordingly.

I am not a fan of big jumps in macros, so I prefer to check progress more frequently (weekly) and make smaller adjustments. If you check progress less frequently, you can add or subtract on the higher end.

If you're stalled on gaining weight, you should add anywhere from 50-150 calories via 10-30g carbs, and 3-5g of fat, depending on your preferences. If you find that not only are you not gaining weight, but you're actually *losing* weight (this sometimes happens with serious ectomorphs whose metabolisms will adapt to pretty much anything to keep them thin), go ahead and make a bigger jump anywhere from 200-300 calories via 50-65g carbs and 5-10g of fat.

Likewise, if you are stalled in a fat loss phase, you can subtract anywhere from 50-100 calories via 10-20g carbs, and 2-6g fat. If you are pretty far into your fat loss phase, and you don't want to drop your calories lower, you can also try swapping 5-10g of carbohydrates for 5-10g of more protein. Increasing protein can help with fat loss through the process of thermogenesis and can increase feelings of satiety.

How do you know if you're stalling in a maintenance phase? In short, nothing is changing. Your measurements aren't changing; your photos aren't changing; your strength is not increasing. At this point, you can either change your goals up to more of a fat loss of muscle building focus, OR you can tweak your macros using the ranges from above. If you choose to tweak your macros (for example, by lowering fat and raising carbohydrates), be sure to give it another few weeks before you determine whether or not it is working for you before you change them again.

UTILIZING RE-FEEDS DURING A FAT LOSS PHASE

Re-feeds can be particularly important during a serious fat loss phase. As we diet, our bodies become accustomed to the lower amount of food, and they start to slow all of our systems down which lowers our metabolism.[29]

As far as your body knows, when you're dieting, you're starving or in a famine. The body, being the badass that it is, tries to protect you from starving to death! This is great for keeping us alive in times of crises (Thanks, body!), but not so great when we want to see our six pack by summer.

As well as slowing down all of your body's functions like digestion and staying warm, little movements like fidgeting, dieting also messes with your hormone levels, including lowering leptin.

Leptin is basically the mother of all fat burning hormones. It is the hormone that sends messages to your brain that you're not hungry and that you're getting enough food and that your body can safely afford to burn fat. These hormonal changes are a major reason why progress in a fat loss phase slows down much more so than in a building phase.[29]

A re-feed is a day when you bump your calories up to maintenance level, lower protein and fats and fill the rest of the calories with carbs. Because leptin responds best to carbohydrates, it is best to focus mostly on carbs during a re-feed day (while still getting essential proteins and fats). [30]

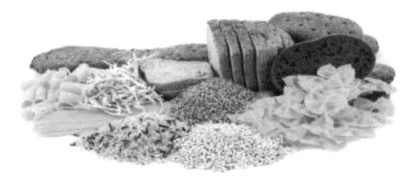

A re-feed day can also be something to look forward to in a dieting phase because you get to eat a larger amount of food than usual, and it's kind of fun! I have also found that re-feed days improve dietary adherence quite a bit when used properly. Consider is a kick-start for your metabolism and the fat burning process.

Re-feeds should be done **in conjunction** with lowering carbs and fats on your other days as explained in the section above. You shouldn't be thinking of a re-feed until at least 4 weeks into dieting or when your progress starts to significantly slow down. You can start with once a week and bump it to twice a week as you become very lean (the leaner you are, the faster your hormone levels drop as your body aims to hold onto your essential body fat[35]).

Try and have your re-feed days on your heaviest training days (usually a leg day).

To set up a re-feed, you increase your calories to maintenance for one day. You also lower your protein and fat to the lowest recommended amounts in the macro calculating section and fill the remaining calories with mostly carbs.

WHEN TO START OVER

Sometimes, you will make so much progress toward your goal that you are almost a different person from where you started! This is usually a good thing! If you find yourself in a situation where you have gained or lost 20 or more pounds, it may be a good time for you to go all the way back to chapter 5 and re-calculate your macros from scratch.

Your body fat and lean body mass is probably quite different from where you started. It is also likely that your metabolic rate has changed significantly. In this situation, re-calculate and start again. This is a good thing - celebrate it!

11 EATING OUT, SOCIAL SITUATIONS AND TRAVELING

Figuring out what to eat when you go out has always been the plight of the vegan, hasn't it? Finding anything that doesn't contain animal products is a challenge in some restaurants. Add flexible dieting into the mix, and you might throw in the towel and say "screw it" for the day. But wait! It can be done!

The most important thing to remember here is that it's called *Flexible Dieting*. You have to be willing to be flexible. You're not going to be able to get everything exactly correct, right down to the gram, but that's okay because you don't eat out every meal of every day of your life, do you? These are often special occasions, meant to be lived and enjoyed, and in the meantime, you do the best you can.

All of the following situations rely on estimating the macros in your meal. This is a skill that requires a lot of practice, so if you don't nail it perfectly from the first attempt, don't worry -- none of us did! It's absolutely key to not just quit - just keep working at it and you will get much better at it!

THE HAND PORTION GUIDE

There is no question that social events require estimation of macros. But one of my favorite ways to do that, is to use a tool that we always have on us: our hands. Now, this is not a perfect system as hand sizes certainly differ, but this is a good way to keep yourself close.

- Your palm represents a portion of a protein food which is about 20g protein.

- Your two cupped hands equal a serving of veggies which is about 10g carbohydrates.

- Your one cupped hand equals a serving of fruit which is about 10-15g of carbohydrates depending on the fruit.

- Your first represents a serving of starchy carbohydrates or beans which is around 30g carbohydrates.

- Your thumb represents a serving of high fat foods like nuts and seeds or avocado and is roughly 10-15g of fat.

- Your finger tip represents a serving of oil, which is about 10g of fat.

Outside of this use your best judgement. For example, you likely know that tofu also contains some fat and beans also contain some protein!

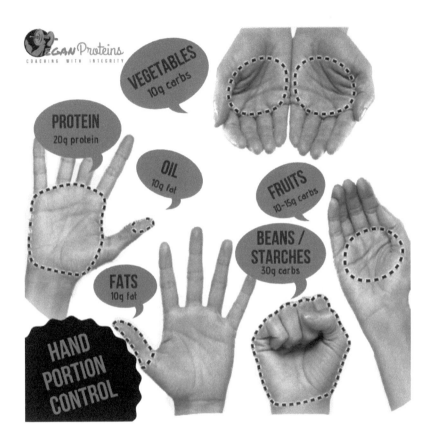

VEGAN Proteins
COACHING WITH INTEGRITY

VEGETABLES
10g carbs

PROTEIN
20g protein

OIL
10g fat

FRUITS
10-15g carbs

BEANS /
STARCHES
30g carbs

FATS
10g fat

HAND
PORTION
CONTROL

EATING OUT

Eating out can be a little bit tricky because unless it's a vegan-friendly restaurant, it's unlikely that they will have much in the way of higher protein vegan foods.

Don't be afraid to look at the menu online ahead of time (many establishments even have their nutrition facts listed online) and narrow down what you'd like to a few options and plan your day around that. You can save some (not all!) of your carbs and fats up for a special occasion, like eating out, because typically restaurant meals are high in both. Determining what you'll eat ahead of time relieves anxiety about on-the-spot food choices. It also keeps you from being *that person* who is logging their food on their phone while everyone else is trying to be social. This is the best option.

More spontaneous trips out to eat can be a little stressful if they take you by surprise, and you will probably have to wing it a bit. Despite not usually having a decent vegan protein option in a lot of places, even chain restaurants often have a veggie burger that happens to be vegan on the menu.

Think about how many macros you have to fill. Do you have a lot of carbs and fat to fill? Then you may be able to have side of fries. Not so much wiggle room? Opt for lower carb options and swap the sides out for steamed veggies or a salad.

Let's pretend that you're in a situation where you choose to order a veggie burger. You ask what kind it is (for two reasons: 1. To make sure it's vegan, and 2. So you can track it more accurately) and it's a Beyond Burger. That's easy to look up. When it arrives, you see it's on a sesame seed bulkie roll, which is also easy to look up (no, it may not be exact, but you will get pretty close). And you get about 1.5 cups of mixed steamed veggies—plug it all in, and you're good to go.

PRO TIP: Unless you order your food with no oil (which you should if you're trying to keep your fat low), just automatically assume that there is anywhere from 10-20g of fat just from oil in your meal. I worked in restaurants for a long time. Trust me on this—the cooks in the back don't care about your macros and they are free pouring oil onto stovetops.

A veggie burger is a pretty easy situation to imagine, so let's look at something a little trickier. How about a stir-fry type bowl with brown rice, veggies, tofu and a sauce of some kind? This has a lot of ingredients and you're not sure how much of each.

You have a couple of options here:

1. Try looking up the restaurant in MFP. You may be surprised to find your meal is already there! That's the best-case scenario.

2. Ask for the sauce on the side and try to estimate how much of each food is in it. Because you've been practicing at home by weighing and measuring your meals, you're getting pretty good at it by now. You estimate it to be 1 cup of cooked brown rice, about 3 oz tofu, another cup of mixed veggies, and when you see the sauce on the side, you realize that it's made mostly of peanut butter. The rest is easy to log; then try looking up "Peanut Sauce" and I bet there will be something close there.

So, you can see, this is not an exact science. As mentioned before however, you need to decide how strict you must be and hold yourself accountable to those standards.

If you're two weeks away from a bodybuilding show, you have almost no wiggle room and need to stick to what you know – like steamed veggies and a salad with dressing on the side.

If you're in a maintenance phase, or looking to put on some size, you are obviously able to take a few more liberties with your food choices.

In certain situations, there is no easy way to look up and track your food, and that can be a bit of a struggle. For example, I often go to a mom and pop flatbread restaurant (read: no nutrition facts to be found anywhere) and order a veggie flatbread with no cheese. There is no way that I can look that up *exactly*. What I have found to be the best way to do this is to look on My Fitness Pal for something from a big chain restaurant that is *similar* to what I actually ate, even if it's not vegan, because I know the macros will be close.

In this particular case, I have found looking up a Domino's Veggie Lover Pizza with no cheese is pretty darn close to what I estimate is in my flatbread pizza.

PARTIES AND SOCIAL SITUATIONS

Social situations, like a party at someone's house, are even trickier. Vegans are already used to not having many options at these gatherings. Since we're already used to these having few options, it may actually be easier for us than it is for many non-vegans.

You can always do the old standby of bringing a dish to the party so that you know you can have it and you know exactly what's in it. As an added bonus, this can also help show other people how delicious and simple veganism can be, which is always a win.

Or you can make the best choices you can by estimating – just like when eating out. One thing I would recommend if you're going to go this route is to get one plate and put what you plan to eat on one plate. It will be much easier to keep track of what you're eating if it's all on one plate rather than eating chips out of a bowl, for example.

I always recommend having some protein before you go or in your bag or car. This way, if they have a protein option, you don't need it and can save it for later. But if they don't, which is more likely, you will not leave so hungry that you reach for the first edible thing you can find.

TRAVEL TIPS

Planning is everything when you're trying to stick to your goals on the road. Do some research about where you're going before you get there so you will have an idea of what kinds of foods you will have access to and what you may need to bring with you.

My absolute number one tip for travel: hit a grocery store. If you're serious about your goals, eating restaurant or gas station meals 3 times a day during travel isn't going to cut it. Nearly every city or town has a grocery store. Here you can easily pick up some healthy, easy to make, or ready to eat foods to stay on track. I do this every time I travel, which is frequently.

Individual protein powder packets are great things to have on you while on the road. They travel well, they don't go bad, and they're pre-portioned. I also like to bring protein bars, vegan jerky, or packets of vegan deli slices or pre-baked and seasoned tofu. The protein bars and jerky don't go bad quickly, so if you don't need them, you don't have to waste them.

Individual oatmeal packets are a great thing to have on the road when you're looking for a nourishing breakfast, and you can even use the coffee pot in your hotel room to make it. Rice Cakes or apples and peanut/almond butter are good travel snacks as well.

Other things I always bring with me when traveling for more than a day are: my mini food scale (depending on how strict I need to be at the time), utensils, napkins, and packets of stevia, my sweetener of choice.

But again, the biggest thing to remember is that your diet shouldn't be ruling your life while you're out with your friends or on vacation. If you are spending more than a few minutes logging or tracking food while you should be living in the moment or enjoying your family, you need to loosen the reigns a little bit (unless you're in contest prep or something similar which requires you to be more strict, in which case I suggest taking your vacation at a different time).

Perfection is the enemy of the good, and you need to focus on doing the best you can, where you are, with what you have. With enough practice at home, and a little planning, all of these situations get much easier.

12 FINAL THOUGHTS

At the end of the day, you have to ask yourself: Can you see yourself eating the way you're currently eating in 5 years? 1 year? 6 months? If the answer is "no" because you're trying to follow a very strict diet to reach your athletic goals, then it is time to re-think your strategy.

I'm not suggesting that you settle for mediocrity and only give a half-effort. What I am suggesting is finding a way to have the best of both worlds. The purpose of life is to live it, and if you're feeling bogged down by an eating style that doesn't allow you to partake in activities you enjoy, then something somewhere will give, whether it's your relationships with your family and friends, your goals, or worse yet, your mental or physical health.

Through the process of learning how to eat flexibly and enjoy special foods in moderation, and without the mental struggle of guilt, you *can* have the best of both worlds a vast majority of the time.

I hope that the end of this book finds you with a new perspective on eating, and at the very least, has opened your eyes to how unhelpful restrictive meal plans and dietary dogma can be for vegans, athletes and humans alike. I would not write about something that I didn't personally believe in and I believe that flexible dieting can be a major tool in ending many people's internal struggles and unhealthy relationships with foods.

It's not always easy, but nothing worth having ever is. You will need to put in effort to make this work for you and your life, but the effort does not have to equate suffering, restricting, and becoming a recluse. You can be strict, without being restricted, and learn to thrive in all areas of your wellness journey.

12 RESOURCES

SAMPLE MEAL PLAN GRAPHICS

These are merely examples of meal plans that could exist using different parameters, tastes, products, meal timing structures, etc. Please just use these as inspiration when building your own plans.

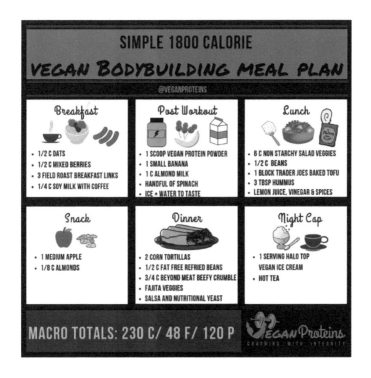

SIMPLE 1800 CALORIE

VEGAN BODYBUILDING MEAL PLAN

@VEGANPROTEINS

Breakfast
- 1/2 C OATS
- 1/2 C MIXED BERRIES
- 3 FIELD ROAST BREAKFAST LINKS
- 1/4 C SOY MILK WITH COFFEE

Post Workout
- 1 SCOOP VEGAN PROTEIN POWDER
- 1 SMALL BANANA
- 1 C ALMOND MILK
- HANDFUL OF SPINACH
- ICE + WATER TO TASTE

Lunch
- 6 C NON STARCHY SALAD VEGGIES
- 1/2 C BEANS
- 1 BLOCK TRADER JOES BAKED TOFU
- 3 TBSP HUMMUS
- LEMON JUICE, VINEGAR & SPICES

Snack
- 1 MEDIUM APPLE
- 1/8 C ALMONDS

Dinner
- 2 CORN TORTILLAS
- 1/2 C FAT FREE REFRIED BEANS
- 3/4 C BEYOND MEAT BEEFY CRUMBLE
- FAJITA VEGGIES
- SALSA AND NUTRITIONAL YEAST

Night Cap
- 1 SERVING HALO TOP VEGAN ICE CREAM
- HOT TEA

MACRO TOTALS: 230 C/ 48 F/ 120 P VEGAN Proteins
COACHING WITH INTEGRITY

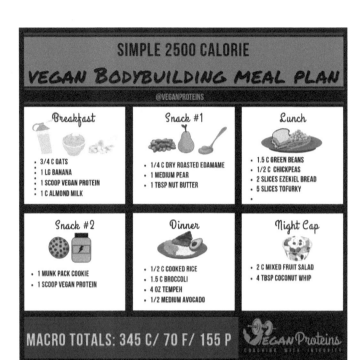

SIMPLE 2500 CALORIE
VEGAN BODYBUILDING MEAL PLAN
@VEGANPROTEINS

Breakfast
- 3/4 C OATS
- 1 LG BANANA
- 1 SCOOP VEGAN PROTEIN
- 1 C ALMOND MILK

Snack #1
- 1/4 C DRY ROASTED EDAMAME
- 1 MEDIUM PEAR
- 1 TBSP NUT BUTTER

Lunch
- 1.5 C GREEN BEANS
- 1/2 C CHICKPEAS
- 2 SLICES EZEKIEL BREAD
- 5 SLICES TOFURKY
-

Snack #2
- 1 MUNK PACK COOKIE
- 1 SCOOP VEGAN PROTEIN

Dinner
- 1/2 C COOKED RICE
- 1.5 C BROCCOLI
- 4 OZ TEMPEH
- 1/2 MEDIUM AVOCADO

Night Cap
- 2 C MIXED FRUIT SALAD
- 4 TBSP COCONUT WHIP

MACRO TOTALS: 345 C/ 70 F/ 155 P

Vegan Proteins
COACHING WITH INTEGRITY

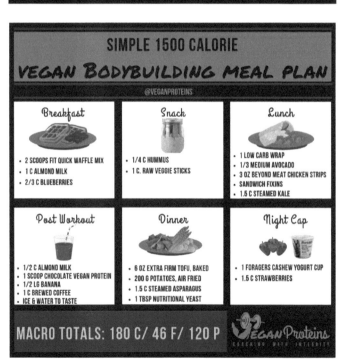

SIMPLE 1500 CALORIE
VEGAN BODYBUILDING MEAL PLAN
@VEGANPROTEINS

Breakfast
- 2 SCOOPS FIT QUICK WAFFLE MIX
- 1 C ALMOND MILK
- 2/3 C BLUEBERRIES

Snack
- 1/4 C HUMMUS
- 1 C. RAW VEGGIE STICKS

Lunch
- 1 LOW CARB WRAP
- 1/3 MEDIUM AVOCADO
- 3 OZ BEYOND MEAT CHICKEN STRIPS
- SANDWICH FIXINS
- 1.5 C STEAMED KALE

Post Workout
- 1/2 C ALMOND MILK
- 1 SCOOP CHOCOLATE VEGAN PROTEIN
- 1/2 LG BANANA
- 1 C BREWED COFFEE
- ICE & WATER TO TASTE

Dinner
- 6 OZ EXTRA FIRM TOFU, BAKED
- 200 G POTATOES, AIR FRIED
- 1.5 C STEAMED ASPARAGUS
- 1 TBSP NUTRITIONAL YEAST

Night Cap
- 1 FORAGERS CASHEW YOGURT CUP
- 1.5 C STRAWBERRIES

MACRO TOTALS: 180 C/ 46 F/ 120 P

Vegan Proteins
COACHING WITH INTEGRITY

SIMPLE 3000 CALORIE
VEGAN BODYBUILDING MEAL PLAN
@VEGANPROTEINS

Breakfast
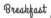

- 1 C NATURE'S PATH GRANOLA
- 1 MEDIUM BANANA
- 1.5 C RIPPLE MILK

Snack #1

- 1/2 C ROASTED CHICKPEAS

Lunch

- 1 C COOKED QUINOA
- 1 C COOKED LENTILS
- 1 C STEAMED VEGGIES
- 6 OZ CUBED SEITAN

Snack #2

- 2 SLICES EZEKIEL BREAD
- 2 TBSP PEANUT BUTTER
- 2 TBSP JAM OR JELLY

Dinner

- 2 C COOKED PASTA
- 1 C PASTA SAUCE
- 1 C COOKED SPINACH
- 1/2 C TVP (IN SAUCE)
- 2 TBSP NUTRITIONAL YEAST

Night Cap
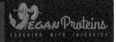
- 1 LARA BAR OF CHOICE

MACRO TOTALS: 425 C/ 70 F/ 170 P
VEGAN Proteins
COACHING WITH INTEGRITY

SIMPLE 1900 CALORIE - GLUTEN FREE
VEGAN BODYBUILDING MEAL PLAN
@VEGANPROTEINS

Breakfast

- 2 SLICES WHOLE GRAIN TOAST
- 1/2 C MIXED BERRIES
- 6 OZ TOFU, SCRAMBLED
- 2 TBSP NUTRITIONAL YEAST
- 1/4 C ALMOND MILK WITH COFFEE

Post Workout

- 1 SCOOP VEGAN PROTEIN POWDER
- 1 SMALL BANANA
- 1 C ALMOND MILK
- HANDFUL OF SPINACH
- ICE + WATER TO TASTE

Lunch

- 1/2 C BEANS
- 1/2 C QUINOA
- 4 OZ TEMPEH
- 1 C COLLARD GREENS
- 2 TBSP BBQ SAUCE

Snack

- 1 MEDIUM APPLE
- 1 TBSP PEANUT BUTTER

Dinner

- 1/2 C JASMINE RICE PILAF
- 2 GARDEIN CHICK'N SCALLOPINI
- 2 C. ASPARAGUS

Night Cap

- CHOCOLATE MOUSSE MADE WITH:
- 6 OZ SOFT TOFU
- 2 TBSP COCOA POWDER
- 1 SERVING CHOCOLATE CHIPS

MACRO TOTALS: 225 C/ 55 F/ 125 P
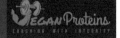
VEGAN Proteins
COACHING WITH INTEGRITY

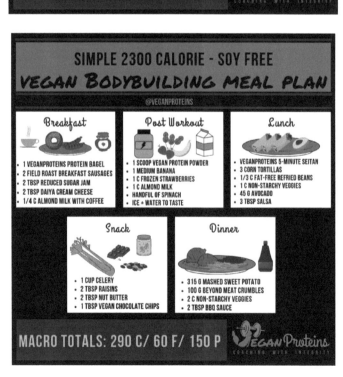

SIMPLE 2100 CALORIE - NO MOCK "MEATS"
VEGAN BODYBUILDING MEAL PLAN
@VEGANPROTEINS

Breakfast
- 60G HEARTSMART BISQUICK MIX
- 30G VITAL WHEAT GLUTEN
- 30G BANANA
- 16G PEANUT BUTTER
- 1/4 C SOY MILK WITH COFFEE
- 50G BLUEBERRIES

Lunch
- 1 BLOCK FIRM TOFU
- 1 C JASMINE RICE
- 2 C NON-STARCHY VEGETABLES
- 3 TBSP TERIYAKI SAUCE

Snack
- 1 SCOOP VEGAN PROTEIN POWDER
- 1 CONTAINER SILK VANILLA YOGURT
- 100G STRAWBERRIES
- 16G ALMOND BUTTER
- 1 TBSP VEGAN CHOCOLATE CHIPS
- WATER TO THIN

Dinner
- 3 OZ EDAMAME PASTA
- 1/2 C MARINARA SAUCE
- 50G SLICE FRENCH BREAD
- 1/2 TBSP EARTH BALANCE BUTTER
- GARLIC (FOR GARLIC BREAD)

MACRO TOTALS: 240 C/ 64 F/ 153 P

Vegan Proteins
COACHING WITH INTEGRITY

SIMPLE 2300 CALORIE - SOY FREE
VEGAN BODYBUILDING MEAL PLAN
@VEGANPROTEINS

Breakfast
- 1 VEGANPROTEINS PROTEIN BAGEL
- 2 FIELD ROAST BREAKFAST SAUSAGES
- 2 TBSP REDUCED SUGAR JAM
- 2 TBSP DAIYA CREAM CHEESE
- 1/4 C ALMOND MILK WITH COFFEE

Post Workout
- 1 SCOOP VEGAN PROTEIN POWDER
- 1 MEDIUM BANANA
- 1 C FROZEN STRAWBERRIES
- 1 C ALMOND MILK
- HANDFUL OF SPINACH
- ICE + WATER TO TASTE

Lunch
- VEGANPROTEINS 5-MINUTE SEITAN
- 3 CORN TORTILLAS
- 1/3 C FAT-FREE REFRIED BEANS
- 1 C NON-STARCHY VEGGIES
- 45 G AVOCADO
- 3 TBSP SALSA

Snack
- 1 CUP CELERY
- 2 TBSP RAISINS
- 2 TBSP NUT BUTTER
- 1 TBSP VEGAN CHOCOLATE CHIPS

Dinner
- 315 G MASHED SWEET POTATO
- 100 G BEYOND MEAT CRUMBLES
- 2 C NON-STARCHY VEGGIES
- 2 TBSP BBQ SAUCE

MACRO TOTALS: 290 C/ 60 F/ 150 P

Vegan Proteins
COACHING WITH INTEGRITY

VEGAN BODYBUILDING MEAL PLAN
1900 CALORIE - "I DON'T WANT TO EAT 6 MEALS" PLAN

@VEGANPROTEINS

Breakfast

- 1 SERVING LAZY GIRL PROTEIN PANCAKES
- 1 LG BANANA, SLICED
- 1 C SLICED STRAWBERRIES
- COFFEE WITH ALMOND MILK

Lunch

- 1 C COOKED BROWN RICE
- 1/2 C BLACK BEANS
- PEPPER, ONIONS, MUSHROOMS
- 1/2 MEDIUM AVOCADO
- 1/2 BRICK TEMPEH
- SALSA TO TASTE

Snack/Dessert

- 1 SILK SOY YOGURT
- 1/2 C FROZEN BLUEBERRIES
- 1/2 C FROZEN CHERRIES
- 1 TBSP SLICED ALMONDS

Dinner

- 1 SERVINGS ONE POT PEANUT NOODLES (LOW CAL OPTION)

FOR MORE RECIPES, VISIT VEGANPROTEINS.COM

MACRO TOTALS: 260 C/ 45 F/ 120 P

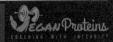

VEGAN BODYBUILDING MEAL PLAN
1800 CALORIE - SOY FREE - GLUTEN FREE - HIGH PROTEIN

@VEGANPROTEINS

Breakfast

- 1/2 C DRY OATS
- 2 SCOOPS BROWN RICE PROTEIN
- 1 C SLICED STRAWBERRIES

Post Workout
- PUMPKIN PIE PROTEIN SHAKE:
- 1 C ALMOND MILK
- 1 SCOOP VANILLA PEA PROTEIN
- 1/2 LG BANANA
- 1/2 C CANNED PUMPKIN
- PUMPKIN PIE SPICE

Lunch

- 2 C COOKED COLLARD GREENS
- 1 C SPICY BLACK EYED PEAS
- 1 SMALL BAKED YAM (150G)

Snack

- 1 MEDIUM APPLE
- 1/4 C ALMONDS

Dinner

- 50G DRY EXPLORE ASIAN PASTA
- 1 C MARINARA
- 1-2 C ROASTED VEGGIES
- 2 TBSP NUTRITIONAL YEAST

Night Cap

- BLUEBERRY CHIA PUDDING
- FOR RECIPE, VISIT WWW.VEGANPROTEINS.COM

MACRO TOTALS: 210 C/ 50 F/ 125 P

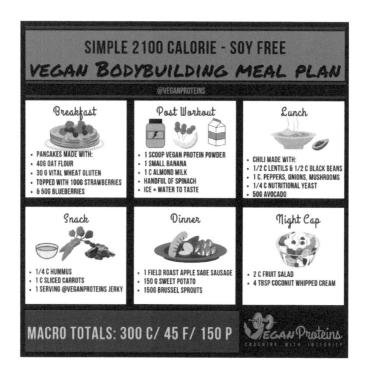

SIMPLE 2100 CALORIE - SOY FREE
VEGAN BODYBUILDING MEAL PLAN
@VEGANPROTEINS

Breakfast
- PANCAKES MADE WITH:
- 40G OAT FLOUR
- 30 G VITAL WHEAT GLUTEN
- TOPPED WITH 100G STRAWBERRIES
- & 50G BLUEBERRIES

Post Workout
- 1 SCOOP VEGAN PROTEIN POWDER
- 1 SMALL BANANA
- 1 C ALMOND MILK
- HANDFUL OF SPINACH
- ICE + WATER TO TASTE

Lunch
- CHILI MADE WITH:
- 1/2 C LENTILS & 1/2 C BLACK BEANS
- 1 C. PEPPERS, ONIONS, MUSHROOMS
- 1/4 C NUTRITIONAL YEAST
- 50G AVOCADO

Snack
- 1/4 C HUMMUS
- 1 C SLICED CARROTS
- 1 SERVING @VEGANPROTEINS JERKY

Dinner
- 1 FIELD ROAST APPLE SAGE SAUSAGE
- 150 G SWEET POTATO
- 150G BRUSSEL SPROUTS

Night Cap
- 2 C FRUIT SALAD
- 4 TBSP COCONUT WHIPPED CREAM

MACRO TOTALS: 300 C/ 45 F/ 150 P

VEGAN Proteins
COACHING WITH INTEGRITY

On the following pages, you will find worksheets to use the formulas in this book more easily.

· DETERMINE YOUR MAINTENANCE CALORIES ·

TRACK WEIGHT FOR A WEEK

Calculate the change in weight over the week.

_____ − _____ = _____

End Weight − Start Weight = Weight Change

HOW FAR FROM MAINTENANCE WERE YOU?

Every pound has 3500 calories, so we can find out how far off maaintenance you've been eating.

_____ X 3500 = _____

| Weight Change | Cals in a pound | Weekly Deviation from Maintenance |

Divide by 7 to get the daily deviation.

_____ ÷ 7 = _____

| Weekly Deviation | Days in a Week | Daily Deviation from Maintenance |

HOW MUCH DID YOU EAT THIS WEEK?

Add up all 7 days of calories and divide it by 7 days to get the daily average.

_____ ÷ 7 = _____

| All 7 days of calories | Days in a Week | Average Daily Caloric Intake |

FIND YOUR MAINTENANCE

Add if you lost weight over the week.
Subtract if you gained weight over the week.

_____ + / − _____ = _____

| Average Daily Caloric Intake | Daily Deviation | YOUR TRUE MAINTENANCE! |

FAT LOSS

Subtract 200-800 from your maintenance calories.

The smaller the deficit, the more likely it is to be just fat lost.

_____ - _____ = _____

Maintenance - deficit = fat loss calories

BODY RE-COMPOSITION

Eat maintenance calories.

Great for athletes for performance, people new to training, people new to flexible dieting.

_____

Maintenance Calories

MUSCLE BUILDING

Add 200-500 to your maintenance calories.

The smaller the surplus, the less likely you are to gain fat.

_____ + _____ = _____

Maintenance + surplus = building calories

3 ▸ **DETERMINE LEAN BODY MASS**

ESTIMATE YOUR BODY FAT PERCENTAGE

Use calipers, a dexa scan, a visual graph such as in this book, or other.

_____ X _____ = _____
Body Weight   Body Fat %   =   Pounds Fat Mass

_____ - _____ = _____
Body Weight   -   Pounds Fat Mass = Lean Body Mass

4 ▸ **DETERMINE PROTEIN GOAL**

Multiply Lean Body Mass by anywhere from .8 – 1.2 to get your daily protein goal in grams.

_____ X _____ = _____
Lean Body   .8 – 1.2   Protein goal
Mass   in grams

Protein has 4 calories per gram, so let's calculate how many calories we're getting from protein. We will need this later..

_____ X   4   = _____
Protein goal   Calories
in grams   from protein

5 ▸ **DETERMINE FAT GOAL**

Multiply Calorie Goal by anywhere from .2 – .4 to get your daily calories from fat.

_____ X _____ = _____
Calorie Goal   .2 – .4   Calories
                                      from fat

Fat has 9 calorie per gram, so we divide by 9 to get the goal in grams

_____ ÷   9   = _____
Calories   Fat goals in
from fat   grams

6 DETERMINE CARBOHYDRATE GOAL

HOW MANY CALORIES WILL COME FROM CARBS

Using the "calories from protein" and "calories from fat" from previous steps, we will determine how many calories will come from carbs.

$$\rule{2cm}{0.4pt} - \rule{2cm}{0.4pt} - \rule{2cm}{0.4pt} = \rule{2cm}{0.4pt}$$

| Calorie Goal | Calories from protein | Calories from fat | Calories from carbohydrates |

FROM CALORIES TO GRAMS

Carbohydrates have 4 calories per gram. So we will divide calories by 4 to get a target in gram

$$\rule{3cm}{0.4pt} \div \quad 4 \quad = \rule{3cm}{0.4pt}$$

| Calories from carbohydrates | | Carbohydrate goal in grams |

7 TIPS

Use the 3 Tiered system when need be. Tracking calories and protein or even just calories is enough for most goals.

Create meal times that work for YOUR life. Ideally 3-6 meals per day.

Give macros at least 4 weeks before tweaking them.

Aim to get around 20% of your daily carbohydrates from fiber and do not neglect micronutrients.

BE FLEXIBLE!!!!!

13 SOURCES

1. Bender, M.M.; Rader, J.I.; McClure, F.D. (1998, March 17) How compliance works -- Title 21 of the Code of Federal Regulations (21 CFR 101.9(g). Retrieved from http://www.fda.gov/Food/GuidanceRegulation/GuidanceDo cumentsRegulatoryInformation/LabelingNutrition/ucm063113 .htm#how

2. Stewart, T.N.; Williamson, D.A.; White, M.A (2002, February) Rigid vs. flexible dieting: association with eating disorder symptoms in nonobese women. Retrieved from http://www.ncbi.nlm.nih.gov/pubmed/11883916

3.Park, M. (2010, November 8) Twinkie diet helps nutrition professor lose 27 pounds. CNN. Retrieved from: http://www.cnn.com/2010/HEALTH/11/08/twinkie.diet.pr ofessor/

4. Young, V.R.; Pellett, P.L. (1994 May) Plant proteins in relation to human protein and amino acid nutrition1'2. Retrieved from http://ajcn.nutrition.org/content/59/5/1203S.full.pdf

5. Norton, L.E.; Layman, D.K.; (2006 February) Leucine regulates translation initiation of protein synthesis in skeletal muscle after exercise. Retrieved from http://www.ncbi.nlm.nih.gov/pubmed/16424142

6. Crovetti, R.; Porrini, M.; Santangelo, A.; Testolin, G. (1998 July 28) The influence of thermic effect of food on satiety. Retrieved from http://www.ncbi.nlm.nih.gov/pubmed/9683329

7. Helms, E. R.; Aragon, A. A.; Fitschen, P. J. (2014 May 12) Evidence-based recommendations for natural bodybuilding

contest preparation: nutrition and supplementation. Retrieved from http://www.jissn.com/content/11/1/20

8. Antonio, J.; Peacock, C.A.; Ellerbroek, A.; Fromhoff, B.; Silver, T. (2014, May 12) The effects of consuming a high protein diet (4.4 g/kg/d) on body composition in resistance-trained individuals. Retrieved from http://www.jissn.com/content/11/1/19

9. Dideriksen, K.; Reitelseder, S.; Holm, L. (2013 March 13) Influence of amino acids, dietary protein, and physical activity on muscle mass development in humans. Retrieved from http://www.ncbi.nlm.nih.gov/pmc/articles/PMC3705323/

10. Lemon, P.W.; Mullin, J.P. (1980 April 1) Effect of initial muscle glycogen levels on protein catabolism during exercise. Retrieved from: http://jap.physiology.org/content/48/4/624

11. Nave, R. Retrieved from http://hyperphysics.phy-astr.gsu.edu/hbase/organic/carb.html
12. Poole, C.; Wilborn, C.; Taylor, L.,;Kerksick, C.; (2010 September 1). The role of post-exercise nutrient administration on muscle protein synthesis and glycogen synthesis. Retrieved from
http://www.ncbi.nlm.nih.gov/pmc/articles/PMC3761704/

13. Pendergast, D.R.; Horvath, P.J.; Leddy, J.J.; Venkatraman, J.T. (1996). The role of dietary fat on performance, metabolism, and health. Retrieved from http://www.ncbi.nlm.nih.gov/pubmed/8947430

14. NIH Curriculum Supplement Series. Retrieved from http://www.ncbi.nlm.nih.gov/books/NBK20371/

15. Horton, T. J.; Drougas, H.; Brachey, A.; Reed, G. W.; Peters, J. C.; Hill, J. O. (1995) Fat and carbohydrate overfeeding in humans: different effects on energy storage.

Retrieved from
http://ajcn.nutrition.org/content/62/1/19.short

16. Donnelly, J. E.; Jakicic, J.; Gunderson, S. (1991 October 12)
Diet and body composition. Retrieved from
http://www.ncbi.nlm.nih.gov/pubmed/1784876

17. Hall, K.D. (2010 March) Predicting metabolic adaptation,
body weight change, and energy intake in humans. Retrieved
from
http://www.ncbi.nlm.nih.gov/pmc/articles/PMC2838532/

18. Hämäläinen, E.; Aldercreutz, H.; Puska, P.; Pietinen, P.
(1984 January 20) Diet and serum sex hormones in healthy
men. Retrieved from
http://www.ncbi.nlm.nih.gov/pubmed/6538617

19. FDA. Title 21, Food and Drugs. Chapter 1, FDA
Department of Health and Human Services. Subchapter B,
Food for Human Consumption. Retrieved from
http://www.accessdata.fda.gov/scripts/cdrh/cfdocs/cfcfr/cfr
search.cfm?fr=101.9

20. Topping, D. L.; Clifton, P.M. (2001 July 8) Short chain fatty
acids and human colonic function – roles of resistant starch
and non-starch polysaccharides. Retrieved from
http://www.ncbi.nlm.nih.gov/pubmed/11427691

21. Kenney, W. L. (2004) SSE #92: Dietary water and sodium
requirements for active adults. Retrieved from
http://www.gssiweb.org/Article/sse-92-dietary-water-and-
sodium-requirements-for-active-adults

22. Lin, P. H.; Aronson, W.; Freeland, S. J. (2015 January 8)
Nutrition, dietary interventions and prostate cancer: the latest
evidence. Retrieved from
http://www.biomedcentral.com/1741-7015/13/3

23. Kollias, Helen. "Research Review: High-Protein Diets – Safe for Kidneys." Retrieved from http://www.precisionnutrition.com/high-protein-safe-for-kidneys

24. La Bounty, P. M.; Campbell, B. I.; Wilson, J.; Galvan, E.; Beradi, J.; Kleiner, S. M.; Kreider, R. B.; Stout, J. R.; Ziegenfuss, T.; Spano, M.; Smith, A.; Antonio, J. (2011 March 16) International Society of Sports Nutrition position and stand: meal frequency. Retrieved from http://www.precisionnutrition.com/high-protein-safe-for-kidneys

25. Campbell, B.; Kreider, R. B.; Ziegenfuss, T.; La Bounty, P.; Roberts, M.; Burke, D.; Landis, J.; Lopez, H.; Anonio, J. (2007 Spetempber 26) International Society of Sports Nutrition position and stand: protein and exercise. Retrieved from http://www.jissn.com/content/4/1/8

26. Phillips, S. M.; Van Loon, L. J.; (2011) Dietary protein for athletes: from requirements to optimum adaptation. Retrieved from http://www.ncbi.nlm.nih.gov/pubmed/22150425?dopt=Abstract&holding=f1000,f1000m,isrctn

27. Stellingwerff, T.; Cox, G. R. (2014 March 25) Systematic review: Carbohydrate supplementation on exercise performance or capacity of varying durations. Retrieved from http://www.nrcresearchpress.com/doi/abs/10.1139/apnm-2014-0027?src=recsys&#.VSxrbxPF9ew

28. Samra, R. A. (2010) Chapter 15 Fats and Satiety. 15. 4. 5. Retrieved from http://www.ncbi.nlm.nih.gov/books/NBK53550/#ch15.r97

29. Trexler, E. T.; Smith-Ryan, A. E.; Norton, L. E. (2014) Metabolic adaptation to weight loss: implications for the athlete. Retrieved from http://www.jissn.com/content/11/1/7

30. Dirlewanger, M.; di Vetta, V.; Guenat, E.; Battilana, P.; Seematter, G.; Schneiter, P.; Jéquier, E.; Tappy, L. (2000 November 24) Effects of short-term carbohydrate or fat overfeeding on energy expenditure and plasma leptin concentrations in healthy female subjects. Retrieved from http://www.ncbi.nlm.nih.gov/pubmed/11126336

ABOUT THE AUTHOR:

Dani Taylor is the co-founder of Vegan Proteins and is a full time coach for vegans who wish to change their physiques, from weekend warriors to professional athletes. She lives in Haverhill Massachusetts with her husband Giacomo Marchese and their four fur babies. She has been vegan since 2002 and has been speaking to dispel vegan myths for nearly as long. She currently competes in the figure division of natural bodybuilding. Dani's passion is helping others realize their full potential in health and fitness with a fully vegan lifestyle, without the nutrition dogma often associated with veganism. She seeks to prove that you can accomplish anything while living a healthy balanced vegan lifestyle. She can be reached at www.veganproteins.com and on Instagram @veganproteins.

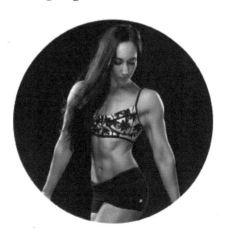